ASSESSING SATISFACTION IN HEALTH AND LONG-TERM CARE

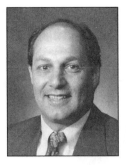

Robert A. Applebaum, M.S.W., Ph.D., is a Professor in the Department of Sociology, Gerontology, and Anthropology and Associate Director of the Scripps Gerontology Center at Miami University, Oxford, Ohio. He has been involved in the development and evaluation of quality assurance systems and long term care system reform for several states. Dr. Applebaum was the guest editor of a *Generations* issue on Quality Assurance, and has published two books on long term care as well as numerous articles and monographs. He has served as a Book Review Editor for *The Gerontologist*, a member of the Gerontological Society of America public policy committee, as co-chair of their task force on long-term care, and as chair of the Social Research, Planning, and Practice section of the Society. Dr. Applebaum holds an M.S.W. from the Ohio State University and a Ph.D. from University of Wisconsin-Madison.

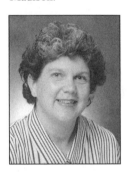

Jane Karnes Straker, Ph.D., is the Director of Policy for the Ohio Long-Term Care Research Project at the Scripps Gerontology Center at Miami University, Oxford, Ohio. Since coming to Miami University in 1993 she has been engaged in applied evaluation research of long term care services and programs for the State of Ohio. She has directed a variety of projects focusing on consumer satisfaction information from over 1,500 nursing home residents and home care clients. She is currently involved in projects examining Ohio's non-certified home health agencies, studying reliability of nursing home MDS+ data and case-mix, and determining cost-effective strategies for collecting consumer information from home-care clients. Dr. Straker received her Master's in Gerontological Studies from Miami University and her Ph.D. from Northwestern University.

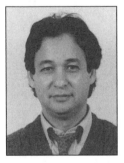

Scott Miyake Geron, Ph.D., is an Associate Professor of Social Welfare Policy and Research at Boston University's School of Social Work. Dr. Geron's research interests include home care and managed care for older adults, quality assurance and assessment, and case management. From 1994–97 he was Principal Investigator of a National Institute on Aging project to develop a measure of client satisfaction for frail elders who receive home-based services, including case management. He is now working with several states and programs in the United States to implement the measure. He was recently guest editor of an issue of *Generations* that focused on assessment from the consumer's perspective. Dr. Geron completed his M.A. and Ph.D. at the University of Chicago. He subsequently completed a two year post-doctoral appointment at the National Long-Term Care Resource Center in the School of Public Health at the University of Minnesota.

ASSESSING SATISFACTION IN HEALTH AND LONG-TERM CARE

Practical Approaches to Hearing the Voices of Consumers

Robert A. Applebaum
Jane K. Straker
Scott M. Geron

 Springer Publishing Company

Springer Publishing Company, Inc.
536 Broadway
New York, NY 10012-3955

Acquisitions Editor: Helvi Gold
Production Editor: Helen Song
Cover design by James Scotto-Lavino

00 01 02 03 04 / 5 4 3 2 1

Library of Congress Cataloging-in-Publication Data

Assessing satisfaction in health and long term care: practical approaches
    to hearing the voices of consumers / Robert A. Applebaum,
Jane K. Straker, and Scott M. Geron.
        p.   cm.
    Includes bibliographical references and index.
    ISBN 0-8261-1305-2 (softcover)
    1. Patient satisfaction.   I. Applebaum, Robert.   II. Straker, Jane K.
III. Geron, Scott.
    [DNLM: 1. Patient Satisfaction.   2. Data Collection—methods.
W 85 A846 2000]
RA399.A1A875 2000
361.1—dc21
DNLM/DLC
for Library of Congress   99-42882
                                                                                CIP

Printed in the United States of America

This book is dedicated to
Bennett, Joshua, Julia, Nicholas, Noah, and Tessa
who remind us each day how important it is to listen.

Contents

Acknowledgments

Many people have helped this book come to fruition. Cheryl Johnson and Betty Williamson provided their magic touch to the text and tables of the manuscript. Our colleagues at the Scripps Gerontology Center, Miami University, and the Boston University School of Social Work provided specific comments and suggestions, but most importantly provided us with a fun and stimulating place to work. Over the past decade, as we have tried to learn about assessing satisfaction, we have subjected many consumers to a range of questions through a variety of data collection approaches. We thank them for their patience and candor in allowing us to learn a little bit about how to hear their voices. Our hope is that older consumers will receive better services as a result.

Part I

Examining Consumer Satisfaction: Context and Methods

Chapter **1**

Why the Growing Interest in Consumer Satisfaction?

Over the past decade there has been a growing interest in consumer satisfaction with products and services. From small human services agencies to large-scale industries, we want to know what consumers think about the services or products provided. At many restaurants, motels, and retail outlets, the consumer can not avoid surveys or questions about the products or services received. Satisfaction surveys from Mr. Goodwrench, Wendy's dad (Dave Thomas), and others in the retail- and services sectors have become commonplace. More recently, health and long term organizations have recognized the importance of consumer feedback. Despite the surging interest in the consumer, providers continually express concerns and frustrations about the lack of adequate tools to gauge accurately consumer satisfaction. This book was developed in response to questions raised about how to assess successfully the satisfaction of health and long term care recipients.

OBJECTIVE AND CONTENT

This book is designed for practitioners, researchers, students, (and anyone else that will buy it), who are committed to hearing from consumers. It originated because of the interest and many questions raised by agency staff and students who were interested in assessing consumer satisfaction. The book is organized into two parts. Part 1 includes background information about assessing consumer satisfaction. Many of the basic questions identified in this chapter will be examined in that section. In Part 2 we present specific chapters based on area or setting. Thus, we include chapters on home care, nursing homes and assisted living, and health care satisfaction approaches. A final chapter will link consumer satisfaction results to service design and improvement.

Our goal is to make this book practical in its application. To this end, we include many examples of questions and approaches used to assess consumer satisfaction. It is our hope that this book allows agencies to enhance their ability to hear what consumers think about the services received and to use this information to improve the delivery of care. It is clear that the search for quality must include data from consumers. Such a search requires both a commitment to hearing from the consumer and knowledge about how best to be successful at providing the consumer with those services. Our objective is to contribute to the knowledge component, but it is almost meaningless if agency and staff are not committed to the hearing part.

Encouraging agency colleagues to share your commitment to hearing from the consumer is a challenging task. As researchers, we have developed our commitment to this area not by someone telling us that this is important, but by having access to information from consumers. When staff are able to view agency programs through the eyes of consumers, and can modify those programs based on consumer feedback, acceptance is generally not a problem. It can be difficult to get agencies to allocate resources to such an effort *apriori*. Organizations have limited resources, and spending staff or dollar resources on research is typically in conflict with the agency's orientation to deliver care. Thus, consumer satisfaction and quality-improvement advocates need to provide examples in order to demonstrate that consumer assessment, quality, and service delivery are inseparable. It is our hope that successful examples will be a common experience for agencies and researchers as they embark on these efforts.

WHY ASSESS SATISFACTION?

The discovery (or rediscovery) of the consumer in the health and long term care arenas has occurred for four important reasons: (1) an increase in competition between health and long term care, particularly as a result of managed care and other capitated funding mechanisms; (2) an increase in public interest in the consumer, including commitments from providers and the government to provide published data on care performance; (3) a growing consumer movement, enhanced by the advocates for people with disabilities who assert autonomy and individual decision making is a key element of quality care; and (4) an increase in popularity of Total Quality Management (TOM), which emphasizes the importance of the customer in achieving quality. In combination, these factors result in considerable interest in gaining input from consumers.

Increased competition in health and long term care has become the hallmark of the 1990s. As a result of almost constant increases in health and long term care expenditures, efforts to control costs now dominate the health and long term care policy debate. Changes in reimbursement mechanisms and the expansion of managed care have developed as system responses to escalating costs. The most notable development on the reimbursement side has been the shift from fee-for-service or retrospective financing systems which pays providers by service, to the implementation of the Medicare hospital prospective payment system in 1983, which provides a set cost per diagnosis, without regard to the actual cost per episode. This system provided an economic incentive for hospitals to reduce the length of stay of patients, and since the advent of the program in 1983, the average hospital stay has been reduced by 3 days (GAO, 1996). Thus, while hospitals want to attract patients to keep their beds occupied, they have an incentive to discharge residents quickly, creating lower occupancy rates. The incentive system has resulted in a paradox, in which hospitals compete intensely for patients so they can discharge them as soon as possible.

A related development has been the growth of managed care. Although many definitions of managed care exist, under most managed care systems a member or enrollee pays a fixed amount per year to a plan, and in exchange receives access to a specified array of health care services. For the aged population, the Medicare managed care provider typically receives the federal Medicare share plus the Part B premium amount. As an added benefit, many of the plans include dental, eye glasses, or prescription drugs; long term care services, however, are not covered. Competition to both attract and keep enrollees is considerable. From an economic perspective, high enrollments are important to ensure solvency. Recent estimates indicate that it costs about $1,000 per individual to enroll a new managed care member. High rates of turnover are clearly expensive, creating a strong incentive for managed care providers to keep consumers satisfied. In addition, beneficiary satisfaction information is publicly available to assist consumers in choosing their managed care plan. These two factors have raised considerably the motivation for managed care providers to assess the satisfaction of enrollees. Financing for other areas of care, including physician services, home health care, and nursing homes, have been or are in the process of being transformed into managed care systems.

Incentives to keep people out of expensive acute or institutional care settings have had dramatic effects on home and community-based services. Over the past 10 years, there has been considerable expansion in the long term care options available to older people with chronic disabilities. In-home care financed through Medicaid, Medicare, and state general revenues, has developed into a large industry as well. Assisted living has seen a dramatic expansion, with extensive private development providing a catalyst for growth across the United States. An expansion of other in-home services and care options, such as adult day care, adult foster care, and respite care, means that there are considerably more opportunities for care than there were a decade ago.

Long term care is changing on the institutional side as well. As a result of the hospital prospective payment system and other managed care initiatives, nursing homes are being used to a greater degree for delivering short-term rehabilitative care. For example, in a recent study in Ohio we found that 47% of those admitted were no longer residents after 3 months, and over 60% were no longer residents after 6 months (Mehdizadeh et al., 1996). The growth in short-stay residents, combined with the expansion of long term care options has resulted in nursing home occupancy rates in the U.S. dropping from 91.8 % in 1985 to 87.4% in 1995 (Strahan, 1997). This puts more pressure on providers to know what consumers need and want.

From the popularity of *Consumer Reports* and Nader's Raiders, to expanded consumer hot lines, to government efforts to publish data on health outcomes for hospitals and HMOs, the Age of the Consumer has become widerspread. There is a growing recognition that consumers of health- and long term care ought to be able to have their opinions heard and have information about the quality of the services or products received.

The concept of having information available for consumers to make an informed choice is not new. For example, the Mobil Travel Guide, designed to get consumers through those relaxing family vacations, has been available since 1958. Having information available for consumers in the health- and long term care field, however, has been a rare occurrence (Geron, 1991). In fact, such an orientation is a 180-degree change from an earlier era, in which the health- and long term care providers were typically unconcerned about providing consumers with information. Under the traditional "expert model", consumers relied on professionals to direct them to the care needed. Data on quality, typically unavailable, was better left to these experts for review. Clients could rely on the health and long term care providers to forward the necessary information.

In the traditional system, information from consumers about the quality of care received was also considered to be not particularly important. Again, the philosophy that the professional was in a far better position to assess quality dominated the provider orientation. The medical aspects of some of the care, the fraility of the consumers, and the attitude that older people (especially those with disabilities) would not want to be in charge of the care received, resulted in a system of care that often ignored the consumer.

Since then, the health care arena in particular has seen a dramatic change in recognizing the importance of customer satisfaction. A recent survey of managed care organizations and hospitals reported an almost universal use of satisfaction surveys. About 33% of these surveys are actually done by outside firms, and the remainder are completed in-house. An indicator of the importance of assessing satisfaction is the growth in customer assessment by private companies. Over 60% of Fortune 500 companies reported surveying and tracking consumer satisfaction with health care covered by company benefits. An additional 21% reported a plan to collect such information in the future (Zimmerman, Zimmerman, & Lund, 1996).

The rise of consumer autonomy is another critical factor contributing to the importance of assessing consumer satisfaction. In both the health and long term care arenas, we are beginning to recognize the importance of consumer choice and decision making on outcomes of care. Health care, with the physician predominantly left in charge of care, and long term care, with its roots in the almshouse (Holstein and Cole, 1996), has long had a health and safety orientation toward care provision. As noninstitutional care alternatives have been expanded for people with disabilities, there has been increased interest in providing consumers with greater choice and autonomy. Led by advocates and people with disabilities, the independent living movement has stressed consumer choice and autonomy as primary values for the long term care delivery system. Under this orientation quality could be achieved only when care providers heard and responded to the consumers' voices.

The consumer choice perspective stipulates that care recipients should be able to have more control over the type of services received and who delivers them. This perspective places a high value on consumer choice. Although health and safety—the two dominant concerns in institutional care—are factors in decision making, these should not be the driving force behind the structure of long term services. The maintenance of the consumer's health and safety, and the expansion of consumer choice and autonomy, are two value systems that are not always complementary in their orientation to care, and may in fact be in conflict. Thus, efforts to regulate quality of care may have to broker between the desire of the consumer to have choice, and the desire of society to guarantee safety. However, if this dillemma is to be resolved, information about what consumers think about the care received will be essential to ensuring quality care.

The emergence of total quality management (TQM) or continuous quality improvement (CQI) is a technique developed to use statistical controls to improve the quality of a good or service produced. Traced back to the work Dr. Edwards Deiming began in postwar Japan, the approach has been credited with improving the production of automobiles and other high technology equipment, first in Japan, and subsequently in the U.S. and other nations. The technique is based on the assumption that if organizations use the resources allocated for inspection and reworking of defective products do it right the first time, they can have higher quality without adding costs. The landmark book by Crosby entitled, *Quality is Free* (1979) is based on that hypothesis.

In our recent studies, we have tried to apply the concepts to health-, housing-, and long term-care services. Since improving quality is the primary motivation for assessing consumer satisfaction, we believe that it is important to view consumer satisfaction as part of an overall quality improvement model. Based on our quality management experiences we have identified five important principles of TOM that organizations need to address in their efforts to enhance quality for consumers:

1. You must know your customers.
2. You must hear the voices of the consumers.
3. Information is essential for sound decision-making.
4. The group is smarter than the individual.
5. Suboptimization is the key challenge facing organizations.

PRINCIPLE #1 YOU MUST KNOW YOUR CUSTOMERS

The first question any provider of goods or services needs to ask is: Who are our customers? Quality management suggests that organizations need to recognize that they have more than one customer. Customers or consumers can be classed into primary and secondary groupings, and can be either internal or external to the organization. For example, in home care the primary customer would be the care recipient, and a secondary customer in a publicly funded program could be a funding or regulatory agency. Internal customers would include agency staff, who receive services from other staff within the organization to do their jobs. External customers in the case of home care could include such participants as care recipients, family members, funding agencies, taxpayers, and regulators. It is important to note that all consumer groups may not have the same needs or requirements. For example, in home care, the range of customers—from consumer, to funder, to regulator—may have very different expectations of the service.

Quality management also recognizes that customers may not always have the same objectives. For example, in long term care we typically see situations where the family would like more hours of care than the direct recipient would. This generally occurs because family members are quite concerned about health and safety issues, while care recipients are generally more worried about protecting their privacy and autonomy in their home. Conflict between consumer groups is normal, and must be recognized. Organizations must make decisions about how to resolve consumer conflict, but first they must know that it exists.

Resolution of consumer conflicts requires an agency's specific response. Such decisions require agencies to balance the needs of various consumer groups. For example, several years ago, at a certain university, such a conflict occurred. The student association had recommended that the university allow condom machines to be placed in the dormitories, in an effort to encourage safe health behavior. The proposal was passed by the student government, by the student housing and health services units, and by the university faculty. But it then went to the university president for final approval—he vetoed it. Why? In this case, the university has a number of customers including students, their parents (who typically pay the bills), the state legislature (who allocates funds to the university), alumnae, and future employers. While the students overwhelmingly supported the proposal, the presidential veto occurred because, in his assessment, the parents' and legislative customers' needs (to assure that students could not possibly be sexually active) were more important than the students' needs (to conveniently purchase condoms). In this example, the organization did not agree on its primary customer.

PRINCIPLE # 2: YOU MUST HEAR THE VOICES OF THE CONSUMER

After identifying the range of customers, the second step is to hear their voices. Historically, health and long term care services have not done a good job of listening to their consumers. In many programs, systematic efforts to ask consumers about the care received was practically nonexistent. Even quality assurance or regulatory efforts typically ignored the consumer. For example, in an effort to ensure the quality of nursing homes during the 1970s and 80s, the federal and state governments developed an extensive survey procedure for assessing the quality of nursing home care. A team of five to ten surveyors would visit a facility for 1–2 weeks to examine quality of care. Prior to the most recent nursing home reform implemented in 1990, the survey process used did not require the review team to talk with any residents of the facility. Such was true for the major efforts used to evaluate health care as well.

All of us have been consumers and understand the importance of expressing our own satisfaction/dissatisfaction with the quality of services provided. But how does the consumer get ignored in such a process? In health and long term care, the consumer gets discounted because there is an assumption that the consumer does not have the expertise to provide useful feedback about quality of care. In contrast, we believe it is essential to hear the voice of the consumer, even when the services may be technically sophisticated. Consumers experience the receipt of services, and their perceived satisfaction or dissatisfaction provides a unique source of information about the quality of health or long term care. The belief that consumers are unable to assess the quality of services has been pervasive among the professional community, resulting in limited experience with assessing consumer satisfaction.

Lessons of quality management from such industries as manufacturing and electronics have highlighted the importance of hearing from consumers. Knowing what consumers want and how they feel about the product or service delivered is critical to quality improvement. How can a program be improved without knowing how those using it evaluate its quality and effectiveness? Without access to information from consumers, efforts to deliver high quality care will remain unsuccessful.

PRINCIPLE # 3: INFORMATION IS ESSENTIAL FOR SOUND DECISION-MAKING

A key principle in TQM is that organizations need good information with which to make decisions. Many health and long term care agencies have limited data on even the most basic descriptive characteristics concerning the clients they serve. Data on demographic, health, and functional characteristics are often unavailable. Other information, such as length of enrollment, reason(s) for termination, length of time it took to receive services, type and amount of services received, and a host of other information, is simply not tracked.

Quality management uses the concept of benchmarking as an improvement technique. Benchmarking—a concept that has been a key component of evaluation research—requires that products or services have performance measures that can be examined over a period of time. Such measures can also be examined across common agencies. Recent efforts to examine nursing facility performance using standardized information collected in the minimum data set (MDS) is an example of such an approach. Carefully designed consumer satisfaction data collected over time and across similar organizations can also be used to benchmark quality performance.

PRINCIPLE # 4: THE GROUP IS SMARTER THAN THE INDIVIDUAL

Although not very popular with CEOs and other high-level managers, this principle states that, in the problem-solving and improvement process, a group will make better decisions than one individual. Related to this idea is the concept that those individuals involved in the delivery and receipt of care must be involved in the monitoring, evaluating, and improving process. This means that information from staff across all levels of the organization, from top administration to direct service workers and consumers, must be received. And it further argues that approaches to improvement should be instituted by working committees, which should include staff from the range of positions within the organization. Information received directly from consumers and employees who have considerable contact with consumers is a key element of this component.

PRINCIPLE # 5: SUBOPTIMIZATION IS A KEY CHALLENGE FACING ORGANIZATIONS

The term suboptimization is one which we rarely use or hear, but the concept is common in agency practice. Suboptimization occurs when one unit within the organization maximizes its own efficiency at the expense of other units. The end result of suboptimization is an overall reduction in organization quality. For example, case management agencies often report that the procurement department will be quite proud of itself for reducing the unit cost for purchased services, only to find out that more case management funds for service monitoring are needed because of poorer quality service provision. Nursing homes report conflicts between the personnel department, trying to recruit new workers and the nursing department, who may feel the new workers are not experienced or qualified enough for the position.

Quality improvement stresses that, rather than having individual objectives or missions, organizations should have one goal—to deliver quality care. Thus, each unit within the organization should have a common goal rather than competing ones. Again, the consumer is the key to this element of quality management. The unifying goal is the delivery of high-quality care to consumers in an efficient and effective manner. To determine whether this goal is achieved requires information on a wide range of areas involved with the delivery of services, with consumer assessment of services being one essential element. Although the consumer is a critical component of quality, it should be emphasized that quality management is broader than assessing consumer satisfaction. Agencies need to develop a quality improvement strategy that involves a range of activities and data-collection approaches. Certainly, an important part of that strategy will involve getting input from consumers about the quality of care received. However, other such data collection must be undertaken under a larger quality-of-services context.

CHALLENGES TO ASSESSING CONSUMER SATISFACTION

Despite the importance of listening to the views of consumers, there are a number of significant challenges to assessing consumer satisfaction. These include training and professional orientation of agency staff, vulnerability and frailty of the population, and difficulties in measurement and data collection strategies.

Training and Professional Orientation. Many professionals in health and long term care are highly trained and their jobs require technical skills. Professional training and expertise are important. However, it is sometimes inconsistent with the idea of listening to the views of consumers. Many professionals believe that consumers do not have the expertise to provide feedback about the quality of care. This results in an orientation in which consumer opinions are not sought or highly respected. As a result many agencies either do not ask consumers for their opinions about the care received or with little interest or enthusiasm. This is a particularly ineffective strategy for the cohort of older people now receiving long term care. Older consumers today do not appear to be as well versed at consumerism as the baby boom generation to receive services in the future. This means that if agencies want to hear from consumers they have to be committed to doing so.

Vulnerability and frailty of consumers. Recipients of care, particularly in the long term care sector, have become increasingly more impaired over the past decade. This is attributable to the increase in the size of the oldest old age group, health care changes that have shifted care from the acute to the long term care sector, and an expansion of long term care options, so that home care and assisted living have become an accepted method of care for highly impaired people. Frailty or impairment poses barriers to the assessment of consumer satisfaction for two reasons: (1) those who are in poor health will be harder to reach and may have difficulties in completing satisfactions assessments (e.g., those with hearing, vision or speech impairments) and (2) physical health has been shown to affect satisfaction responses, so that those who are more disabled are more likely to express more dissatisfaction. Cognitive impairment among consumers also represents a challenge to assessing satisfaction. Both the institutional and in-home care settings are serving an increased number of consumers with some form of dementia. This means that it is becoming increasingly more difficult to get input directly from all consumers.

Measurement and data collection. Asking consumers about the quality of services is a difficult task. Health and long term care services are by nature personal, which means that each consumer will have different expectations about the nature and quality of services. Actually, health care is both personal and technical. Sometimes consumers may not know if the care is being delivered properly. Sometimes the proper care is not what the consumer wants. The development of a valid and reliable measure is doubly complicated by data collection issues. Those include both the client frailty issues discussed above, but also cost and operation issues faced by agencies. Most agencies have experience in only the delivery of services, not research data collection. Issues about *how, who, what,* and *where* plague efforts to assess consumer satisfaction. Should agencies hire outside staff to implement such an effort; use their own employees, develop their own instruments, collect information via mail, telephone, or in-person methods? How many consumers does an agency need to hear from, how much should this cost, how often should it be done? There are numerous technical issues faced by agencies and researchers attempting to implement consumer satisfaction efforts. In many cases, researchers don't agree on the answers, making agency decisions on strategy that much more difficult.

The remainder of this book is designed to help agencies and researchers address these challenges, as they strive to hear the voices of the consumer. We are well aware that the road blocks to success are numerous. However, the outcomes of listening to consumers, and ultimately improving the services delivered, provide benefits that make such an effort an important organizational investment.

Chapter 2

Theory of Consumer Satisfaction

By definition, consumer satisfaction with services is largely defined by the nature of the service, program, or treatment that is the subject of evaluation. Satisfaction measures a consumer's affective response to a service or provider. Many analysts however, suggest that this is only one component of satisfaction and that the construct of consumer satisfaction includes a range of dimensions. This chapter will review the basic theory of consumer satisfaction, describe the multidimensionality of the construct of satisfaction in long-term care, explore the importance of expectations in making satisfaction assessments, and describe the relationship between consumer satisfaction and quality of services.

THEORY OF CONSUMER SATISFACTION

The satisfaction literature is extensive, but there is surprisingly little discussion in long-term care about the psychological and cognitive processes that lead to satisfaction responses. Most of the theoretical and empirical work has been done in product and marketing research, which is keenly interested in how consumers evaluate the performance or quality of products and services, and how such evaluations affect subsequent consumer behavior (Yi, 1990). In this literature, consumer satisfaction has been variously defined as a cognitive assessment between expectations for a service and how the service is experienced, an affective or emotional response to services received, or a combination of the two (Davies & Ware, 1988; Pascoe, 1983; Attkisson & Zwick, 1982; Aharony & Strasser, 1993). The predominant theoretical model in the past 10 years is based on what is called the "expectancy disconfirmation" model (Yi, 1990; Rust & Oliver, 1994). While not a pretty turn of phrase, it is fairly descriptive.

In this paradigm, satisfaction results from: (1) a cognitive evaluation of the perceived performance or quality of the various attributes of a service compared to expectations about those attributes; and (2) an affective response to that evaluation. Satisfaction (or dissatisfaction) with a service occurs when there is a "disconfirmation" between expectations and actual performance. Satisfaction occurs when actual performance exceeds expectations; dissatisfaction occurs when the client's experience with a service falls below expectations.

Figure 1 depicts a conceptual model of client satisfaction. Generally, there is wide agreement in the literature on general components of the model, although there is intense debate about the direction of some of the effects between the constructs shown. For example, Pascoe (1983) and others have shown that affective responses also may be based on the reaction of the consumer to the immediate experience of a product or service (shown in the figure by dotted lines). Others have documented that expectations directly affect satisfaction. As satisfaction research continues, more complicated versions of the model are also being developed. For example, analysts have proposed a variation in which satisfaction is a function of perceived quality and disconfirmation when disconfirmation occurs, and a function of expectations when disconfirmation does not occur (Anderson & Fornell, 1994).

A related issue discusses how well the model applies to the evaluation of satisfaction with a service such as long-term care that is received over time. The "expectancy disconfirmation" model is based on a single reaction or postconsumption experience of a product, although analysts have extended the model to consider a consumer's ongoing evaluation of a service over time (Anderson & Fornel, 1994). For example, the development of the SERVQUAL instrument, a multi-item measure of service quality, is based quality as a cumulative construct or overall assessment of a firm's service delivery system (Parasuraman, Zeithaml, & Berry, 1985).

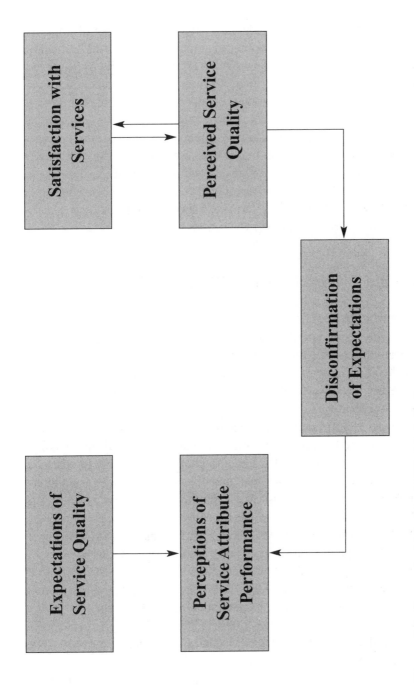

Figure 2.1 Conceptual Model of Client Satisfaction

From this brief discussion of satisfaction theory a number of implications are apparent for the assessment of satisfaction with long-term care services. The importance of the consumer's experience with or perceived quality of the service, product or item suggests that any satisfaction instrument of a long-term care service must encompass the attributes or dimensions of long-term care considered important to consumers. A second implication concerns the importance of expectations in satisfaction assessment. Expectations are an important antecedent of satisfaction that serves as a baseline against which the perceived quality of a service are compared and also have an independent and direct effect on satisfaction. How to determine the dimensionality of long-term care services and consumer expectations will be addressed in next two sections.

THE DIMENSIONALITY OF SATISFACTION

A considerable body of health care research that has examined patient satisfaction with physician-administered or acute care. Early explorations of the dimensionality of patient satisfaction indicate that client satisfaction with health care is a multidimensional construct. In one early study, Ware, Davies-Avery, & Stewart (1978) reviewed over 100 studies on patient satisfaction and identified the following major dimensions in the content of available survey instruments: interpersonal manner of provider, technical quality of care, accessibility-convenience, finances, physical environment, availability, continuity, and efficacy/outcomes of care. Other researchers have also found that patient satisfaction encompasses technical and interpersonal aspects of care, access to and continuity of care, and physical setting (Cryns, Nichols, Katz, & Calkins, 1989; Cleary & McNeil, 1988; Lebow, 1974;). Overall, however, there is little consensus about the specific number, type or relation of dimensions across locations or types of care (e.g., hospitals vs. HMOs; nursing care vs. physician care) or within a specific locus or type of care. Methodological issues also have been found to affect satisfaction responses. For example, research has shown that different conceptualizations and measurement approaches (e.g., direct versus indirect) produce very different patient satisfaction ratings (Roberts, Pascoe & Attkisson, 1983).

The application of these findings to long-term care warrants a strong caveat. Health care research in acute care settings is not a good guide for the use of or client satisfaction measures in long-term care. Long-term care is different in many respects from acute or office-based health care (Kane, Kale, Illston & Eustis, 1994). Compared to the circumscribed episode of a physician visit or acute medical episode, the time horizon for long-term care is elongated or even ongoing. The health problems of a long-term care recipient involve a consumer's daily living situation and tend to be not only enduring but complex and multiply determined. Because long-term care is a living situation of long or even permanent duration, the quality of life of the older person also becomes a matter of monitoring and assessment. Moreover, while long-term care does sometimes require the use of sophisticated technologies, much of the service is "low tech," often provided by personnel with limited training and without professionally derived standards of practice.

One general problem found with measures of client satisfaction currently available is the lack of precise definitions for satisfaction with long-term care services. Because words like "satisfaction" or "satisfied" may have different meanings to different consumers (Gutek, 1978), the involvement of the consumer is necessary to ensure that a measure fully represents the dimensions of quality considered important to service recipients (Riley, Fortinsky, & Coburn,1992; Geron, 1998a). Unfortunately, most available studies are based on researcher or provider perspectives, and not the older recipients of services. Equally important, even when consumers have been involved in the development of a measure (Woerner & Phillips, 1989), the perspectives of minorities have been absent. The inclusion of minority perspectives in the development of a client satisfaction measure is essential to obtain a measure that assesses the full dimensions of satisfaction as defined by the multiethnic consumers of these services (Geron, 1998b; Jackson, 1989).

Findings from research on client satisfaction of frail older persons with home care that was based on consumer defined notions of satisfaction, including the perspectives of ethnic minorities, confirm that the construct domain of satisfaction with long-term care services is constitutively different from that of acute care (Geron, 1995). From analysis of focus group discussions with African-American, Hispanic and Caucasian, we found that satisfaction with long-term care services is a complex and multifaceted concept, encompassing multidimensional attributes that are similar to but different from those frequently identified in the literature on satisfaction with acute or medical care. Satisfaction with home care services, like heath care, is based on assessments of the technical competence, reliability and interpersonal characteristics of workers; however, individual choice, advocacy of workers, and adequacy of services—issues not identified in the literature on acute care satisfaction—were also viewed by consumers of home care services as important dimensions of home care service satisfaction.

EXPECTATIONS

The "expectancy disconfirmation" model highlights the importance of understanding consumer expectations in satisfaction assessments. According to Oliver (1981), "expectations are consumer-defined probabilities of the occurrence of positive and negative events if the consumer engages in some behavior". Expectations are an essential antecedent of satisfaction that serves as the subjective standard against which the perceived quality of a service is compared, and also have an independent and direct effect on satisfaction.

But not all expectations are the same. Miller (1977) was one of the first satisfaction researchers to delineate a typology of expectations, making distinctions between ideal, minimum, expected, and deserved expectations. The ideal or desired level of performance represents what the consumer believes the quality of service should be and serves as a maximum standard. In contrast, a minimum expectation for quality is the lowest level anticipated. A predicted or expected level of performance is based on averaging past experience(s) and comparing actual performance to what is predicted to occur. Asking the consumer to consider equity and costs in determining the level or quality of performance involves a deserved level of service.

Because of these differences in types of expectations, most satisfaction researchers believe that to measure satisfaction, it is necessary to establish which type of expectation is used by individual consumers in making their satisfaction assessments (Pascoe, 1983). Besides individual differences, expectations for care can vary culturally (Sheer & Luborsky, 1991) and may be affected by length of service, class, and other factors (Linder-Pelz, 1982; Rust & Oliver, 1994). The influence of setting on the recipient's expectations may be particularly problematic for older adults residing in institutions, where "learned dependency" may alter expectations enough to make otherwise unsatisfactory care appear to be satisfactory to respondents (Geron, 1991).

To establish a common standard, satisfaction assessments should state what type of expectation from service recipients is to be used as the basis for making satisfaction responses. Here, clarity in stating the standard is essential. Asking consumers to use expected or predicted performance as a basis to inform satisfaction assessments about actual performance can be complicated in long-term care. While most service recipients of nursing home–or home care have no prior experience with receipt of the type of formal services associated with these settings prior to their need for care, almost all have performed similar services themselves (e.g., bathing, eating, dressing, and so on) or seen others perform them. Folke (1994) notes that past experience, one common basis for developing expectations about future service performance, may be based on direct experience by the consumer or anecdotal experience as reported by others, and may be influenced by written records, comments from other consumers, and memory.

Some instruments explicitly address the issue of expectations. For example, the SERVQUAL instrument (Parasuraman, Zeithaml, & Berry, 1986) contains an expectations section of the survey constructed with reference to an ideal company that delivers excellent quality of service. A second section contains evaluations of actual performance of a specific company. As such, instrument is framed within the standard of ideal expectations, and the instrument is a deliberate comparison of actual to ideal performance. In some situations, the assessment of expectations can occur prior to conducting the satisfaction assessments; that is, before the consumer has begun receipt of services. However, in many cases, retrospective determinations of expectations can be made.

SATISFACTION AND QUALITY

Consumer satisfaction is often considered synonymous with service quality, but there are important differences between the two constructs. Satisfaction scores do not necessarily translate into quality ratings, as the following examples illustrates. Suppose two similar groups of consumers receive the same type of service. Suppose further that the two groups are similar demographically and have been found to hold similar expectations for the quality of services that will be provided. If, using a valid and reliable measure, significant differences in mean satisfaction are observed between the two groups, is it reasonable to assume that the quality of service received by the consumers who express more satisfaction is higher than the quality of service received by the consumers who expressed less satisfaction? The answer is no, because of distinctions between satisfaction responses and service quality.

The most important difference is that quality dimensions are necessarily service-specific, while satisfaction assessments are not. Quality assessments must relate to the nature of the service evaluated. The quality of a restaurant's meals, for example, could be assessed by examining the technical quality of the meals (the freshness of the ingredients, the diversity of the menu, the skills of the cook or cooks in preparing the meals, the temperature of the meals served, and so on). It would be unfair to assess the quality of meals by assessing the ambient noise level, wait-time and politeness of the serving staff, or the price of the meals. Satisfaction assessments, however, can result from any dimension of a service considered important to consumers, quality-related or not. These can include not only non–food related items like those already mentioned, but can include factors not at all under the control of the restaurant, including crime in the neighborhood, noise from a construction project next door, or expensive parking. It is this difference that suggests that satisfaction is a broader concept that service quality because quality is one of the service dimensions considered by consumers in making satisfaction judgments.

Another important difference between satisfaction and quality is that quality judgments can be formed without experience, but satisfaction assessments are necessarily based on actual experience. The quality of many products or services can be assessed by reputation or reviews. For instance, one could reasonably form quality judgments on cars, computers, or stereophonic equipment by reading evaluations in consumer magazines or technical reviews. However, one couldn't properly say one is satisfied or dissatisfied with a product or service without using or directly experiencing the product or service.

To return to the example, poorer satisfaction assessments may not mean that the quality of services is substandard. That is likely to be the case, or even probable, but it is not certain. All that is certain is that the consumers in one agency are less satisfied with the same service than are consumers of another agency. To determine why will require an investigation of services provided in both settings. It may be that the more dissatisfied consumers actually receive services that are as good or better than those provided to the more satisfied consumers, but are responding to service system issues affecting the delivery of services that may be beyond the control of the service provider; for example, turnover rates among staff and providers, problems of arranging services in rural or urban areas, and so on. To conclude, consumer satisfaction with a service is an indicator, but only one indicator, of service quality, and the reverse is also true: service quality is one factor, but only one factor, used in making consumer satisfaction assessments.

CONCLUSION

This chapter has reviewed the theory of satisfaction, and some of the issues involved in making satisfaction assessments and interpreting satisfaction assessments. Satisfaction involves a comparison of expectations to perceived or experienced attributes of a service, which underscores the importance of using consumer-derived notions of satisfaction to develop service satisfaction instruments. This definition of satisfaction also suggests that public policy has a role in shaping satisfaction responses, by helping consumers to have clear expectations for the services they will receive.

Chapter **3**

Approaches to Measuring Consumer Satisfaction

If you've read this far, you're probably convinced that gathering input from consumers is something that you should do, but also something that cannot be approached the same way in every situation. Assessing consumer satisfaction with services is somewhat like cooking—there are a million ways to do it, and all of them produce results with subtle (or not so subtle) differences. The goal of the next two chapters is to describe the basic ingredients of the consumer satisfaction assessment, so that you can develop an approach that best fits the needs and resources of your organization. In this chapter, we examine what questions to ask and explore different approaches to collecting data from consumers. In chapter 4, we discuss how to select consumers for study and how to examine results.

As we discussed in chapter 1, the first step in approaching the measurement of consumer satisfaction is to decide who your consumers are. Managed care companies and insurers, employers who purchase insurance for their employees, government agencies that purchase services through Medicare or Medicaid, individual consumers or residents and their families and friends all may have a stake in and an opinion on their satisfaction with those services.

Ultimately, however, the primary customer of interest is the person who actually uses the service. Managed care companies and insurers want their customers to be satisfied with the services available through their health plans. Employers want satisfied employees—health benefits are a costly portion of operations, and when employees are dissatisfied with the services received under those benefits monies might be better spent on contracts with a different provider. Government agencies increasingly view enrollee satisfaction as an important component of quality care, along with service cost and outcomes. Families have an important stake in feeling that their relatives are adequately cared for, but their satisfaction may be affected by different factors than those of the actual recipient of services. Despite concerns that consumers and families do not know enough about the technical aspects of care to make informed judgments about quality, they do know how they feel about the care they are receiving. Their input lets providers know where they need to improve, and also provides information for potential consumers who are making choices about purchasing services in the future. Consumer input can be used as one indicator of service quality supplemented by input from staff, consultants, and others who can provide technical expertise. The strategies for measurement discussed here are those for assessing the satisfaction of primary consumers, and in some cases, secondary consumers such as families and friends. How this information is used is ultimately up to the service provider, payer, or other purchaser of services.

Ultimately, the questions you choose to ask, the approach you use for asking them, the number and kind of consumers you ask, and the way you use your findings are determined by a number of choices and constraints. Survey data collected from a large sample of consumers are no substitute for actually observing care or talking with individuals. On the other hand, individual stories do not substitute for input from many. There are those who say that all attempts to gather information about a subjective phenomena such as "satisfaction" will ultimately result in frustration. However, with an understanding of the limitations of different strategies, one can make an informed choice about the kind of information that can be obtained from a particular approach, as well as a realistic determination about the kind of information that will not be obtained.

WHAT DO WE WANT TO ASK CONSUMERS?

As discussed earlier, satisfaction has a number of dimensions, some of which may be more or less salient to different consumers. The most important rule of thumb for determining what domains of satisfaction are worth assessing is to begin by seeking consumer input. Individual consumers know a lot about the services they receive, how well they are working, and what aspects they find most and least satisfying. If, for example, resident councils are of low interest or value to nursing home residents, their satisfaction with the operation of the resident council is unlikely to color their perceptions of the facility overall. On the other hand, if meals are highly important, this is an area that must be included in order to capture overall facility satisfaction. Visitor parking and visiting hours are probably not important issues for nursing home residents, but could be expected to affect family members. Meister and Boyle (1996) found differences among current residents, current residents' families, families of deceased residents, and staff, regarding the extent to which different domains were perceived as being important to quality of care. The staff and families of deceased residents thought that interpersonal issues were most important; families of current residents valued the technical aspects of care, and current residents valued technical aspects, interpersonal issues, and attributes of the setting equally. In order to apply satisfaction results to service improvement, input from a variety of groups will produce the best overall picture of care.

Assessment of consumer satisfaction needs to examine both objective and subjective aspects of the service. Objective questions are useful for providing quality indicators, particularly when the domains covered are those related to outcomes. On the other hand, technical aspects of care may be secondary to consumer satisfaction with interpersonal relationships between the provider and the consumer repeatedly having an effect on overall service satisfaction. Many surveys combine subjective questions, such as "Overall, how satisfied are you with the services you receive?" or "Are you treated with dignity?", and objective items like "Do your workers arrive on time?"

Small-scale approaches, in which one probes deeply into the care situations of a few individuals, and large-scale approaches, in which one asks questions the same way across a large number of individuals, necessarily result in different kinds of information. Each approach has its merits and is useful for producing different kinds of information. A combination of small-scale and large-scale approaches provides complementary information, as well as illuminating the different results that are obtained when only one approach is used (Reinharz & Rowles, 1988). The best recipe for a useful assessment of consumer satisfaction is one that incorporates several data-collection strategies so that one approach may make up for the limitations of another.

Some information about satisfaction can be gleaned from a systematic examination of information that you may already have on hand. Minutes of resident council meetings, areas mentioned in suggestion boxes, complaint logs, and incident reports, can inform you on which areas of your organization are strong and those areas that need improvement. This type of information can be a helpful starting point to begin thinking about what to cover in a customer satisfaction study.

SMALL-SCALE APPROACHES TO ASSESSMENT OF SATISFACTION

The approaches covered in this section generally rely on gathering in-depth information from a small number of people. Often referred to as "qualitative methods," small-scale approaches allow us to examine individual feelings, to examine why clients react as they do, and to explore the world of the care/service recipient. What it means to be a service recipient, the meanings attached to the receipt of care, and the values one places on different actions and aspects of service, can all best be explored in small-scale studies. Such approaches include focus groups, observation, and individual interviews. Small-scale approaches are also valuable for exploring variations among ethnic groups and socioeconomic strata.

Focus Groups

Focus groups are a particularly economical approach for gathering information when one wishes to explore a large overall question. Focus groups with frail elders may be particularly challenging because of the number and type of disabilities of the participants. The number of participants should be from 7 to 10, so that everyone can see and hear the conversation. Each group usually lasts about an hour, although when participants tire, it may be best to cut the group short. Quine and Cameron (1995) suggest a length of 30–45 minutes for groups of disabled elders, and also suggest that 5 or 6 participants as an optimum number. Extra participants should be recruited in case of illness on the day the group is held. Special attention should be given to providing comfortable seating and a quiet area for the group. Because travel is often a problem for people who experience disabilities, transportation should also be provided. Offering such support to participants removes one reason for nonparticipation and ensures that participants arrive on time. When possible, compensation for the group members' time should also be provided. This is one way to impress upon participants the extent to which you value their opinions. Where monetary compensation cannot be provided it may be possible to get contributions of gifts or services from local businesses, which can be passed on to focus group participants.

Focus groups are led by a facilitator whose main task is to keep the group on track while allowing the group conversation to go into unforeseen topics or areas. In addition to the facilitator, a note taker should be on hand to take brief notes of the ongoing conversation, particularly to identify different participants' input. Groups should be tape-recorded and transcribed for later examination. Participants should be provided with information about the purpose of the group and should be asked for signed written consent for their participation and recording.

The group often begins with a "grand tour" question such as, "I'd like each of you to tell me a little about the kind of help you get from Agency A". After everyone has had an opportunity to speak, follow-up questions can be used to draw out particular kinds of information. For example "Mr. X, you said that you like the homemaker you have now better than the one you used to have. What is it about the one you have now that you like better?" When these types of probes have been exhausted, a new group question can be asked. A set of questions for discussion is used by the facilitator, but the group determines the extent to which each topic is covered. For example, if the group has a great deal to say about the way meals are provided they may discuss the types of foods offered, the temperature of meals, and, where applicable, the ambiance of the dining room, their relationships with their dining partners, and even the comfort of the dining room furniture. On the other hand, if the group has little to say about a topic little time should be spent. Information from focus groups provides a good basis for determining which aspects of care should be covered in a more quantitative survey, and also provides information that may aid in interpreting survey results. Quantitative surveys may provide information about which aspects of care are more satisfying than others; information from focus groups may help us to understand why those differences are observed (Merton, 1987). A strength of focus groups is the way in which group interaction produces insights which might not be found without the interaction of the group (Packer, Race, & Hotch, 1994). The group process may also elicit some strategies for improvement. Sharing opinions with others and being part of the group may reduce anxiety for some older adults. In addition, participants may respond to another's reported experiences with very different experiences of their own. This allows the researcher to gather information that might not have arisen without the group dynamic. Groups often end with a "round-robin" summation, in which each participant is asked to state what he or she thinks is the most important information the group has covered. This activity ensures that everyone has a chance to share their opinions, and also helps the facilitator put the entire discussion into perspective.

More than one focus group should be conducted on the same topic. Sometimes groups take on a personality of their own because one or two participants lead the discussion and influence the group in directions that participants might not normally have found worth pursuing. This last caveat is particularly important given Merton's warning that focus groups are not designed to be a substitute for quantitative data, nor are they designed to be reliable or valid. That is, we cannot presume that the issues raised by a group of clients from the Loving Care Home Care Agency represent the range of patterns and types of responses that would be elicited in a focus group of clients, either from the same agency or another similar type of agency. In addition, those who can be enticed to participate in a group conversation may not be those who actually have strong opinions about their care. One can picture the very dissatisfied client who, nonetheless, would never dream of airing his or her complaints publicly. One of the most important roles of the group facilitator is to encourage all members to participate equally. One can keep a group on target with a specific set of questions that are developed ahead of time.

Focus group participants can be recruited to elicit a broad range of viewpoints. One might recruit a group of participants from all those who had complained about their services, a group from informal caregivers of clients, a group of new clients, a group of long-term clients, or any other type of consumer grouping relevant to the questions one is interested in answering.

As previously mentioned, focus groups are a relatively economical way to gather information, but they are not without costs. A focus group study completed with clients in different locations of Ohio cost, on average, about $500 per group. This included travel expenses for the facilitator and the note taker, snacks and drinks for the participants, transportation costs for the participants, and a payment of $15 to each participant.

In-Depth Interviews

Individual interviews are a second strategy for gathering information from consumers. Interviews may be conducted in-person (generally preferable for interviews with people experiencing a disability), or over the telephone. These individual interviews can provide a supplement to issues raised in focus groups, or can replace the focus group as a way of initially exploring satisfaction issues. Merton believes that focus groups grew out of the practice of focused interviews—a technique designed to identify the aspects of one's experience that explain the outcomes observed in quantitative studies. As with focus groups, the reasons for satisfaction and dissatisfaction can be explored. The advantages of individual interviews are several: they allow clients to express themselves more honestly in a one-on-one setting; they remove some of the difficulties that those with hearing, speech, or other types of impairments, may have when interacting in a group; and they can explore the issues of an individual in greater depth than would be possible in a group interaction. Arranging transportation for participants, finding a time that works for all participants, and finding a suitable room or public facility to accommodate a group meeting are all focus group problems that are alleviated by conducting the individual interview. On the other hand, one can conduct a focus group with eight participants or conduct one interview in about the same amount of time. Gathering input from a similar number of respondents is more costly in individual interviews.

Individual interviews can be used on their own or as a second step in measure development. Recurring themes, which suggest important aspects of satisfaction, can be quantified into larger-scale satisfaction studies. The first step might be to hold several focus groups which explore issues of consumer satisfaction, and then analyze the transcripts to identify common themes regarding influences on satisfaction. From these groups, a set of open-ended questions can be developed. Individual interviews can help in wording questions appropriately, provide information about the range of responses that will later be developed into response categories, as well as information about the relevance of questions. In individual interviews, questions can be reworded and reasked until the respondent understands them. Answers can be probed until they are clear. These are activities that cannot be easily accomplished with a focus group and which are invaluable in preparing a quantitative consumer satisfaction survey.

Observation

One method for understanding the dynamics of satisfaction is to observe how services are delivered. Observations are usually conducted with small numbers of people, but often occur over long periods of time. Observation as a strategy for collecting information about consumer satisfaction requires the observer to become an active viewer of the interactions between service provider and recipient. Although one may look daily at what goes on around him, becoming a research observer involves nonjudgmental recording of appearances, actions, and reactions. Over time, and with continued observation, one can begin to draw conclusions about the meanings behind observed behaviors.

Of necessity, an observer should be an outsider. The care provided in front of a co-worker or supervisor may be quite different from that provided when an outside observer is present. Ethically, employees and clients must be informed that the observer is conducting research. Observing over a long period of time allows the observer to "fade into the woodwork" and care provision becomes more like what would be provided when one is not observed. One member of our research team spent time observing in a large Medicaid nursing home by working in the resale shop and assisting the activity director. Over time, she moved from outsider to insider status as she learned resident and employee names, learned her way around the facility, and exhibited a general understanding of the organization. Residents' satisfaction or dissatisfaction with their care was evidenced through facial expressions, conversations with caregivers, compliance or noncompliance with requests, and in direct comments to the observer. We learned a great deal about satisfaction that the administrator could have used to improve services, as well as employee and resident satisfaction. In another study, we spent 3 months observing the home care provided to 6 clients. The length of time allowed us to observe changes in both the client and providers, the development of relationships, the informal negotiations around how care is provided, and it allowed us to understand care provision and receipt as a dynamic, evolving process. Observing 30 clients for one day, another legitimate small-scale approach, would provide very different information about home care.

One may structure one's observations to include only specific kinds of information. One could observe interactions between aides and residents, and "ignore" everything else that is going on. One can conduct observations during different shifts, on weekends and weekdays, or in different areas of a facility. Traveling with one home care service provider provides a different viewpoint than staying with one client. The strategy chosen varies according to the type of information one is most interested in.

Recording of notes on a daily basis is an essential part of observation. Complete details of what occurred, as well as verbatim conversations, should be recorded if possible, and judgments or conclusions about their meaning should be avoided. In the analysis phase, judgments can be made about meanings based upon the entire observational record. Translating or summarizing a conversation loses the participant's common language; these words and terms could be useful in constructing structured measures later on (Spradley, 1980).

Observation is time-consuming and labor-intensive. In our experience, 4 to 5 hours of note writing may be required for every 2 to 3 hours of observation. Using a tape recorder for notes and having them transcribed later is a possibility, but one that adds greatly to the cost of such a project.

When residents or clients are cognitively impaired and are unable to report on their care, observation is an excellent strategy. Observation may also be a strategy for describing how care is provided. It can be used at any time during the assessment process. For example, observation of the care provided in Wing A and Wing B might provide some explanations if these residents showed differences in a structured satisfaction survey. Observing the care in Wing A and Wing B might also provide information that would be useful in developing a structured satisfaction survey. Opening your facility or agency to students at a local college or university might be one effective way to incorporate an observational strategy into an overall examination of consumer satisfaction.

Diaries and Written Records

Diaries consist of having customers record, at regular intervals, their opinions or objective facts about the services they received. Long-term care consumers can be asked to report about the services they got that day and how well those services were delivered. How was the food today? Was it hot? Did you have a choice of things you liked? Did the dietary aide/meal-delivery person treat you with respect? Was the meal on time? Is there anything else you would have liked that wasn't included? The advantage of the diary approach is that it recognizes that everyone has bad days—both providers and clients. It helps to account for those days by giving us a picture of average service. Several different strategies can be used to administer the diary/record-keeping approach. Brief surveys can be delivered along with the meal on a meal tray for immediate completion, when the homemaker comes to visit, or a weekly "log" can be delivered periodically for consumers to fill in every day and return when it is completed.

LARGER-SCALE APPROACHES

Using a Quantitative Measure

As the following chapters will discuss, a number of consumer satisfaction instruments are available. While satisfaction instruments for health ser-

Table 3.1 Selecting a Measure

Available Measures . . .	Original Measures . . .
allow for comparisons with benchmark data or across providers	do not provide comparability with other services
usually have published reliability and validity	require that reliability and validity be established
do not require input from researchers/methodologists	require time and expertise to develop
may not be directly applicable for a particular provider	can tap unique aspects of service or areas of particular interest
do not require pretesting when previously used with a similar sample	require extra time and expense for pretesting and revision

vices are plentiful, other areas are more limited in the availability of existing instruments. Chapters 5, 6, and 7 provide some suggestions on available instruments, and how to evaluate and adapt existing instruments for your own use. When deciding whether to use an existing instrument or to develop a new one, consideration should be given to a series of questions. As shown in Table 3.1, using an existing satisfaction measure allows service providers to compare their facilities and services with others using the same measure (if data from others can be located). Existing measures usually have previously established validity and reliability and they do not require input from researchers or methodologists, resulting in a lower cost. On the other hand, they may not address all areas of interest, or may address services or issues that are not applicable. If an existing measure must be adapted, then the advantages of reliability and validity, comparability across providers, and lower needs for time, money, and expertise no longer hold true. When a provider has a specific area of interest, designing an original measure can be worth the time and effort required for measure development. If, for example, plans were underway to reorganize the structure of case management in an agency, it would be worthwhile to examine satisfaction with case management in-depth both before and after the change, to determine whether it impacted clients in the hoped-for way.

The information gathered from focus groups and/or individual interviews provides an important source of data regarding instrument choice or development. Focus groups provide information about the words and phrases people use to describe their experiences (O'Brien, 1993). They also provide important information about the relevant domains that influence satisfaction. If existing instruments do not "fit", in terms of meaningfulness to clients and the needs of the organization for service improvement, choosing to develop an original measure may be the best solution.

Quantitative measures ask the same questions of respondents in the same way, and usually ask respondents to choose their answers from a set of response categories. A good satisfaction measure contains items that fully describe the attributes of consumer satisfaction. A single-item measure such as "Overall, how satisfied are you with the services you are receiving?" is not recommended (Geron, 1998). Most satisfaction measures use many items to cover a wide range of service areas and facets of each service. Responses on each service can then be summed into a scale. Multiple items increase reliability and validity, and when favorable and unfavorable statements or questions are asked, they are useful in preventing individual tendencies to agree, regardless of item content (Geron, 1998).

Responses often use a Likert format; that is, a range of responses that can be rank-ordered from most positive to most negative. Table 3.2 shows some typical response options for satisfaction measures. If you want to be able to tell prospective consumers that "90% of our homecare clients rank our service as good or excellent", then a quantitative measure with structured responses would be useful.

Items should be brief, clear, and address only a single topic. Asking "How satisfied are you with your homemaker's kindness and respect toward you?" is asking two questions. The homemaker might be very kind, to the point of being patronizing or condescending, and therefore not very respectful.

Approaches to Information-Gathering

Consumer input regarding services can be obtained through a variety of approaches. The most commonly used are written surveys (administered

Table 3.2   Typical Response Options for Satisfaction Measures

Satisfaction	Evaluation	Frequency	Agreement
1 = Very satisfied	1 = Excellent	1 = All of the time	1 = Strongly agree
2 = Somewhat satisfied	2 = Good	2 = Most of the time	2 = Agree
3 = Neither satisfied nor unsatisfied	3 = Fair	3 = Sometimes	3 = Neither agree nor disagree
4 = Somewhat unsatisfied	4 = Poor	4 = Rarely	4 = Disagree
5 = Very unsatisfied		5 = Never	5 = Strongly disagree

Sauce: Adapted from Geron, 1998.

either by mail or distributed in person), telephone interviews, or in-person interviews. All three strategies can provide quantitative information suitable for producing numeric satisfaction scores. Such information is valuable when comparing facilities, services, or even health plans. The limitation of surveys, however, is their lack of explanatory information. For example, we may gather information that tells us that nursing home residents in Wing A are more satisfied with their care than the residents of Wing B. Unless we already know a great deal about differences between Wing A and Wing B, we may be unable to say why these satisfaction differences exist. This limitation is where a background of information from focus groups or interviews can aid in interpretation of results. Another strategy is to supplement quantitative forced-choice responses with open-ended questions. A question can be directed to those who chose a dissatisfied response by asking them to briefly explain why they were dissatisfied or what caused their dissatisfaction. This approach can also provide valuable information for applying results to quality improvement. On the other hand, it increases the length and difficulty of the questionnaire and may increase the number of people who fail to complete the questionnaire to the end. Trade-offs such as these are the hallmark of consumer satisfaction research.

Table 3.3 Selecting a Survey Mode

	Advantages	Disadvantages
Self-administered	Lowest cost; allows respondent to complete at own pace; guarantees anonymity or confidentiality; may get most honest responses	Lowest response rate; literacy required; vision and writing ability required; may be difficult to convey complex topics
Telephone interview	Mid-level cost; can use appropriate probes to ensure validity of responses; can be longer and/or more complex than self-administered survey	Costs increase if consumers require toll calls, more tiring than personal interviews, difficult to compensate for impairments, sample limited to those with phones
Face-to-face interview	Can collect the most complete information, can observe and/or collect environmental information; can be used with most impaired recipients	Costly, time-consuming; respondents may give socially desirable responses

Table 3.3 compares the three most frequently used data collection methods on a variety of factors. As shown, often, the major limitation in conducting consumer satisfaction surveys is cost. In-person interviews are the most expensive, telephone interviews are next, and written self-report surveys are the least costly method. In a recent face-to-face interview study, we followed a group of long-term care service consumers for a period of 2 years and conducted face-to-face interviews with them. At the first contact, when we had fairly good information about phone numbers and addresses, we spent about $60 per completed case for face-to-face interviews. After 2 years, when we spent more time trying to track down respondents (calling directory assistance, contacting caregivers regarding the whereabouts of their family member, etc.), our per-case data collection costs came to $75. This included the time spent to reach respondents by phone to schedule an interview (or to find a new number when a phone number was unlisted or a letter was returned), drive-time to the interview, mileage reimbursement, and the actual time spent conducting the interview. Additional costs include mailing a precontact letter to let them know that they will be contacted for an interview, telephone bills for pre-interview contacts, wages for data entry, and data analysis. Often, the budget is the main deciding factor in the method that is chosen.

Before beginning to conduct in-person or telephone interviews, intensive training for the interviewers is required. This training ensures that all interviews will be administered in the same way. Even experienced interviewers need training on the particular instrument they will be administering.

Self-Report Surveys

Written self-report surveys generally collect quantitative information that allows respondents to choose their answers from a set of response categories. Two of the main advantages of self-report surveys are their low cost relative to other methods, and their relatively quick output compared to interview methods. Written self-report questionnaires can be distributed at the same time, while interviews may be conducted over a longer period. Written surveys ensure that all questions are asked in the same way of all respondents, and allow respondents anonymity and confidentiality. Self-report questionnaires generally alleviate the problem of social desirability often found in interviews; that is, respondents give a more honest response than they might to an interviewer, particularly on sensitive questions. Some data may also be more accurately obtained through a written survey—respondents may take the time to check their calendars or gather information they would have guessed at or estimated to accommodate the time pressure of an interview.

Self-report surveys have a much lower cost due to the little amount of time required to administer them. Our estimates suggest that they cost as little as one-third of the cost of administering a telephone interview. Where surveys can be distributed and collected without mailing, the cost is even lower.

However, when one is working with a frail population (e.g., clients of long-term care services) self-report surveys often pose their own problems. Written surveys can be intimidating and complex. In addition, those with vision problems or difficulty writing may find a written survey impossible to complete. However, the literature suggests that when a survey is of direct interest, older people do show a high level of cooperation in completing and returning questionnaires.

Cost estimates should include printing and mailing the survey, followed by a postcard reminder to those who have not completed and returned the survey within 2 weeks. A second questionnaire mailing after the reminder further encourages those who have not completed their questionnaires to return them. This method of follow-up increases the response rate and broadens the sample. Those who must be encouraged and reminded to participate may differ in some important ways from those who comply at the first request (Brambilla & McKinlay, 1987). Any cost increases are offset by our ability to obtain a representative sample of respondents.

Telephone Interviews

Telephone interviews are more costly than self-report surveys, are about half the cost of face-to-face interviews, and have several advantages which may make them particularly useful. Individuals with vision impairment and difficulty writing can easily participate in a telephone interview. Hearing impairments do not necessarily prohibit one from participating in a telephone interview, given the wide availability of telephone amplifying equipment. Telephone interviews allow the interviewers to clarify unclear answers to make sure they understand; they also offer the respondents the opportunity to clarify the questions they are being asked. Because of the possibility to explore both questions and answers, one's trust in the data collected is likely to be higher. For example, McHorney, Kosinski, and Ware (1994) found that mailed surveys had significantly more missing data than the same surveys administered over the telephone. When different sets of questions are to be asked depending upon some response category, telephone interviewers can negotiate the questions to be skipped and reduce the complexity of a similar written survey. One study reports comparable data quality obtained from mailed surveys, telephone interviews and face-to-face interviews (Herzog & Kulka, 1989).

One important consideration in determining whether a telephone interview is appropriate for your consumers is their level of frailty. Face-to-face interviews allow for the establishment of rapport between the interviewee and the interviewer and may be less stressful. Older adults may be quite sensitive to the pace of an interview, and telephone interviews generally move more quickly than face-to-face interviews; a cause for concern when interviewing older respondents who experience disability. Telephone interviews provide only auditory information, while face-to-face interviews can incorporate written materials or visual aids, and mailed surveys can be completed at a pace most comfortable for the respondent. In a comparison of telephone interviews and face-to-face interviews, older respondents were more likely to ask how much longer the telephone interview would take and therefore rate it "lengthy," even though the face-to-face interviews actually lasted longer (Herzog & Kulka, 1989). This suggests that a lengthy survey instrument would best be administered in-person.

Another important consideration is the availability of phones in your population. Excluding those without phones might exclude large numbers of nursing home residents, or the poorest among your home care clientele.

In-Person Interviews

While some researchers assert that face-to-face interviews are the method of choice for interviewing older adults, others assert that this method is not always justified, particularly where time and money are limited (Herzog & Kulka, 1989). Doing something is probably better than doing nothing if you cannot afford face-to-face interviews.

For some kinds of information, face-to-face interviews provide the only alternative. For example, information about the client's environment, their ability to perform specific kinds of tasks, and their reliability as an informant can best be assessed in-person. For persons with cognitive impairments, in-person interviews can elicit valid information in a way that telephone interviews or written surveys cannot. Researchers who compared reports of dysfunction between self-administered questionnaires and face-to-face interviews found that the self-administered version only captured 45% of client impairments, while the face-to-face method accurately captured 86% of the impairments. On the other portions of the survey, however, correlations between the two methods were .98 or higher (Anderson, Kaplan, & DeBon, 1989). It is unclear how the two methods would compare on surveys of satisfaction with services.

Like telephone surveys, face-to-face data collection allows interviewers to probe unclear answers and allows respondents to ask for question clarification. A further advantage is that they allow for the development of rapport between interviewer and interviewee. Response rates to in-person interviews are generally higher than for other modes (Gold & Wooldridge, 1995), perhaps due to the added value attributed to the personal interaction.

In-person interviews allow interviewers to use visual aids (for example, cards with response categories printed in large print, or pictures of faces for responses to how one feels about a particular issue). They also allow respondents to use communication boards, for respondents with hearing impairments to read along with the interviewer, and for other alternative communication methods. These may be particularly important for some groups of older clients.

Face-to-face interviews may also have some disadvantages as well. As previously mentioned, they are costly. One of the criticisms of assessing client satisfaction with services is that older people depend upon those services and are reluctant to voice criticisms. Face-to-face interviews can only promise confidentiality, but mailed surveys can offer anonymity, or at least an increased perception of anonymity. Where interviewers would have to be recruited from volunteers, or others known to service recipients, this issue is particularly salient.

In-person interviews are also more likely to suffer from biases due to social desirability. The downside of the rapport established between interviewee and interviewer is that the respondent often tries to give the "right" answer or present their "best" side in order to impress or please the interviewer. This behavior may result in interview data that are less reliable and valid than data that were collected via another method. This behavior also speaks to the importance of using "outsiders" as interviewers. Even volunteers that have only a limited association with your organization may affect the responses of your residents and clients. While it is possible to use volunteers as interviewers, training will be a critical factor in collecting objective data.

CONCLUSION

This chapter has outlined some of the approaches for assessing consumer satisfaction. Ultimately, the choice of strategies is influenced by expertise, time and cost constraints, and the kind of information that the organization needs. No one strategy will be right for every organization, and it is quite likely that a combination of strategies will be more helpful than relying on only one approach. The next chapter looks at some issues involved in implementing a consumer satisfaction strategy, including choosing participants, recording data, and working with consultants.

Chapter 4

Implementing a Consumer Data Collection Strategy

In the previous chapter, we examined the many approaches available to agencies to collect information from consumers. Now we will look at some technical questions about implementing the satisfaction strategy. Who should be selected for study? How many consumers are needed to provide confidence in the data collection approach? When is it okay not to talk with consumers directly? How do we decide on the right strategy for our agency? And finally, what do we actually do with this information?

WHO SHOULD WE TALK TO?

Sample Size

One of the most frequently asked questions regarding consumer survey information is "How many people should we survey?" Unfortunately, the answer is always the same: "It depends." For the several "small-scale" approaches covered in chapter 3, the general rule-of-thumb is to keep interviewing or conducting focus groups until you reach redundancy; that is, until the amount of new information you are gathering with each interview or group is minimal. Redundancy might be reached after three focus groups or ten interviews; but you might also need to continue, when time and budget permit. The focus is on in-depth information, rather than obtaining results that are representative of all consumers.

In order to appropriately determine sample size, for larger-scale approaches researchers consider the type of statistical analyses that will be done, the level at which their findings will be viewed as significant, and the acceptable degree of accuracy. By determining the answers to these questions one can actually calculate the exact sample size necessary for each item in the survey (Blalock, 1979; Kraemer & Thiemann, 1987). With samples that are too small for the type of statistics to be performed, one runs the risk of mistakenly accepting one's results as valid when they are actually due to chance, or rejecting one's results as due to chance, when they are actually based on cause. As a rule-of-thumb, the larger the sample size the less risk of error. On the other hand, each person included in a sample costs money—the determination of sample size is a trade-off between obtaining accurate results and conducting a satisfaction assessment that is affordable. With fewer responses, it is likely that real or significant effects may be missed; with very large sample sizes almost anything will be significant.

A helpful strategy may be to think in terms of a percentage of your clientele. However, in this approach, the proportion actually sampled will vary by the size of the agency. For example, for agencies with more than 1,000 clients, 10% of the client base may represent a good sample size. For organizations with 500 clients, 20% of the client base would provide fairly accurate input. Agencies that may serve 150 clients may need to survey 33% of their clientele in order to gain a representative sample. In general, for studies that are looking for statistical significance, close to 100 clients would be a reasonable minimum. Many of the issues related to sample size depend upon the way the information will be used. To provide proof to a funding agency that a demonstration program to retrain nurse aides results in increased resident satisfaction, statistical significance is important. If your goal is to use information internally to improve performance, substantive significance is more important than statistical significance. You can best decide whether to pursue the issues that make the residents of Wing A half of a percentage point more satisfied than the residents of Wing B. This result could be found to be statistically significant, but meaningless to you in terms of your ability to intervene or otherwise apply this information to daily practice.

The other factor affecting which sample size to select is the response rate you expect to achieve. If you expect that 60% of your clients will return their mailed surveys, and you need at least 100 responses for the type of analyses you would like to do, then you should draw a sample of 170 names.

Sample Selection

Hand-in-hand with the issue of sample size is the issue of sample selection. The best sample is one that is representative of the entire population of consumers. One of the first issues in sample selection is developing an accurate listing of the population. For ongoing clients, this is probably a fairly simple task; when one wishes to survey past clients or their families, more attention must be given to determining the population. Should we include clients who were active in the last year? In the last 6 months? Where an outside evaluator is involved, how can we keep client names and addresses confidential? Several strategies can help to answer these questions. In developing a population that includes previous clients or residents, recall is an important issue. Recall for very specific kinds of information is fairly limited and you would do well to limit your population to current or very recent clients. On the other hand, more general types of satisfaction questions are probably easily answered by clients as long as 6 months after they have stopped receiving services. If you have conducted some small-scale work with previous clients this can guide your choices on the type of questions that people are able to respond to over varying periods of time. Clients are likely to be able to give objective information, such as the number of times providers were late, for only a few weeks; they may be able to provide subjective information, such as whether they were treated with respect, for a longer period of time.

Generally, we offer clients confidentiality but not anonymity. In other words, we know who our respondents are, but we never analyze the data with the intent of identifying a particular person, nor would we make identifying information available to the service organization. We often place a code number on the questionnaire, which is then tied to a list of names.

Knowing something about your respondents allows for additional types of analyses. You can compare the satisfaction of residents in Wing A with those in Wing B, or across different home care providers in a case management agency, or different physicians in a managed care practice. You may wish to link interview data with client assessment data, and compare satisfaction among clients with different levels or types of impairment. Although you may record information such as age, gender, place of residence, disability level, etc., as part of the satisfaction survey, using information you already have available keeps your surveys (and the time required to collect and record the data) shorter. It also allows you to do more in-depth analyses. If you use a code number in a visible spot on a written survey, you should explain how that code number will be used, such as to "identify those who have already returned their questionnaires so they will not receive a reminder mailing".

In order to conduct your satisfaction assessment, you will have to contact your sample of clients. The initial contact is usually made by a letter which explains the purpose of the satisfaction assessment, describes how results will be used, provides some information regarding confidentiality, and offers clients the option of refusing to participate.

Often, concerns are raised about clients being contacted by an outside evaluator. How can we protect our clients' confidentiality while allowing outsiders to have access to client names, addresses, and phone numbers? One approach is to have those who are willing to participate indicate their willingness by returning a postcard or contacting the evaluators, and to then draw a sample from these willing participants. We believe that this strategy is unacceptable because it is likely to result in a small and nonrepresentative sample. As previously mentioned, there may be something quite different about those who are willing to participate when first asked, and those who respond after two or three follow-ups. A better strategy is to add a statement about program evaluation as part of the information release materials that new clients and residents must sign. A local case management agency includes the following statement in their enrollment materials: *I give my permission for AGENCY to provide my name, address, and telephone number along with information about my service needs to those providing services and those evaluating the services that I receive.* Clients are aware that the agency will evaluate services under such an approach. Announcements via direct mail, newsletters, bulletin board postings, or flyers handed out by service providers can let all of your clients know that a customer satisfaction survey will be conducted. Using this strategy can help allay client concerns about confidentiality. An agreement which establishes a legal linkage between the evaluation agency and your agency can help to protect your organization as well. Establishing a contractual relationship with an evaluator establishes a right to information in the same way that direct employees of your organization have access to client information. Those who are later contacted to participate are also more likely to participate if they understand the importance of the endeavor; they may even feel lucky to be one of "the chosen".

There are also ways to limit client exposure—sampling can be done with client identification numbers without providing any further information on the client population not included in the sample. Whatever your approach, staff at the evaluating agency and in your organization should be prepared to answer questions about the survey, discuss concerns with clients, and provide reassurances about the process. Every contact mailing we send to clients results in phone calls from clients who have additional questions and concerns not addressed by the contact letter.

Almost every evaluator will agree that choosing participants at random is essential to the accuracy of results. In a true random sample, every person in the population has an equal likelihood of being selected and each combination of individuals has an equal chance of selection (Blalock, 1979).

Before choosing a random sample from all consumers, researchers consider whether they want to make generalizations to all of their consumers or whether they need information from particular subgroups or types of consumers. A nursing home corporation might be interested in several levels of data that determine the size and composition of their sample. They may need information from only one facility, which could be gathered from a sample of consumers and families from that facility. They might need state or regional level data, in which case they need a random sample of residents from facilities in that state or region. They may need information from all of their facilities in which case a random sample of residents from all of their facilities should be surveyed. Samples can be stratified, that is, designed to be representative of the larger population in important ways. Consider a corporation that has 500 facilities which they manage. There may be differences between their large and small facilities, their urban and rural facilities, or the facilities that they own and those they manage. If one randomly drew resident names from all of the facilities, by odds, more residents of the largest facilities would be surveyed than would residents of smaller facilities. If most facilities were urban, then more urban residents would be surveyed. If the sample is to be representative of all consumers, then these odds result in a sample that reflects the population. On the other hand, if there are important differences between subgroups, stratifying the sample ensures that each group has enough members in the sample in order to do meaningful analyses. Before choosing to stratify a sample, one should be clear about the reasons behind the sample stratification and the kind of information and comparisons that stratification will allow.

The best way to choose a truly random sample is to put all of the consumers names into a file, arrange them in a random way (perhaps by the last four digits of a phone number or other nonmeaningful method), then begin selecting with the nth consumer based on a beginning point chosen at random from a table of random numbers. Some statistical programs, such as SPSSx (Statistical Package for Social Sciences) can read database files, arrange cases at random, as well as sample at random. If one knows the percentage of clients that need to be sampled, one can easily choose every tenth or twentieth client for inclusion in the sample.

The advantage of this strategy is that the sample is truly representative of the whole population of consumers. The disadvantage is that a number of clients will be unable to participate in the study because of cognitive impairments or physical disabilities. One often-used strategy is to develop lists of those able to be interviewed, or able to complete a questionnaire, and draw a sample from these lists. This strategy, while convenient, should be avoided since it does not provide an equal opportunity for all types of residents to be included. Our preferred solution is to draw a sample from all clients and to get input from those who are unable to participate themselves by using friends or family members as proxy respondents.

USE OF PROXIES

In general, proxies are used when clients are unable to complete a questionnaire or participate in an interview for reasons of physical functioning–or cognitive limitations. In the case of a long-term care service population, proxies may be necessary for a high number of consumers. For example, in our study of applicants for long-term care services, proxies were necessary in approximately one-third of the cases. Magaziner (1992) suggests that, in health surveys of older people, about one-fifth of those in the community and half of those in nursing homes may be unwilling or unable to participate. Given the importance of including the viewpoints of frail and impaired consumers along with their more robust counterparts, we recommend the use of proxies.

Using proxies, however, is not without its problems. Do proxies consistently report lower or higher levels of satisfaction than would be obtained if we talked to the respondents themselves? Research suggests that there is better respondent/proxy agreement on objective rather than subjective questions. However, if proxies do not consistently report higher or lower than their respondent counterparts, we may assume that the reporting errors are occurring at random and will not consistently influence your results one way or another. Another strategy, when large numbers of clients are cognitively impaired, is to collect all of the data from proxies. This ensures that any biases occur in the same way for all clients. This differs from surveying family members directly, however. As previously mentioned, the issues of importance to families are not necessarily the same issues that are important to clients and residents. One type of data would be based on what families think their relatives would say, the other asks them to report what they think directly.

Usually, however, proxy reports are combined with information gathered directly from consumers. How do we decide which clients should be contacted directly and which clients should be included by proxy?

1. *Develop a consistent screening strategy to determine which clients in the sample may be unable to participate themselves.* In nursing homes, MDS (Minimum Data Set) assessments provide clinical indicators for cognitive impairment, verbal abilities, and whether a guardian or a Power of Attorney exists. Depending on the level of difficulty of your questions, you may want to have less or more stringent indicators of cognitive impairment. As you will see in the following chapters, some questionnaires and survey instruments have been successfully used with cognitively impaired populations. Home health agencies have assessment data that generally includes

cognitive impairment data as well. Unfortunately, a diagnosis of Alzheimer's is not a clear indicator of an inability to participate; information about short-term memory and decision-making ability is better suited to determining which clients should be included by proxy.

2. *Determine whether your survey or interview instrument can be adapted to compensate for other kinds of impairments.* Providing a written copy of the interview questions and responses for respondents to follow in interviews can compensate for hearing impairments. Recruiting volunteers to assist residents in completing questionnaires may allow some participants to be included who would otherwise be unable to participate.

If clients are clearly too impaired to participate, even with adaptations of your instruments, the next step is to use proxy respondents. The following caveats will assist you in collecting valid and reliable data from proxy respondents.

1. Adapt contact information, such as letters and flyers about the survey for proxies. Letters can be changed from "you have been chosen to participate" to "you have been chosen to respond on behalf of your *relative*".

2. Determine that a particular care giver, guardian, or other proxy, is actually the best person to speak for the respondent. Often, the primary contact listed on service agreements may not be the person who best knows the client. Before conducting an interview with a proxy, make sure that he or she feels well qualified to speak about the opinions of the client.

3. Adapt the questionnaire or interview instructions to include frequent reminders that the proxy is speaking on behalf of another. For example, the instruction "Tell me which answer most closely matches your opinion", would be modified to read "Tell me which answer you think most closely matches your RELATIVE's opinion". Frequent reminders throughout the survey can help proxy respondents keep on track with what they know to be their relatives' opinions, vs. what they think themselves.

WHAT DO I DO WITH MY INFORMATION?

The level of detail you want from your information will determine the type of analysis software needed. We typically conduct all of our analyses using SPSSx, but there are other options. This allows us to examine questionnaire items for statistical significance, to control for other variables, such as client-disability level, while examining differences in satisfaction or significant predictors of consumer satisfaction. On the other hand, if average scores on a question or the number of respondents for each answer is enough to meet your needs, a spreadsheet or database program could be enough. In our concluding chapter, we will discuss additional strategies for analysis and the ways in which you can use different levels of information.

Each question must be given an identifying name or number, and answer categories should also be provided with corresponding numbers. "Yes" or "no" can be recorded or coded in your spreadsheet as "1" or "0". "Excellents", "goods", "fairs" and "poors" become "4s", "3s", "2s" and "1s". Designing the coding system and preparing for data entry is an important step, since this will ensure that you obtain the kind of results you need.

WHO SHOULD DO MY CONSUMER SATISFACTION ASSESSMENT?

The size of your budget, the expertise of your staff, and the amount of time you can devote to a consumer satisfaction study are all important considerations when deciding whether to hold an assessment inhouse or hire an outside evaluator. Outside evaluators have several advantages over inhouse employees: (1) they are perceived to provide the most unbiased information, (2) they have the staff and expertise, and (3) they have the ability to compare your results with other facilities for whom they have also conducted satisfaction surveys. On the other hand, outside evaluators can be costly.

A hybrid approach combining insider and outsider evaluation might involve consultation with a researcher regarding the research design, including mode of administration, sampling, and data entry. Fielding of the survey (mailing, telephoning, interviewing, observing, conducting focus groups, or distributing logs) could be conducted inhouse by volunteers or students (staff is a last resort). Data could be entered inhouse, with reporting and analysis provided by the outside evaluator.

Often, a chain of facilities or another kind of organizational group collaborates on a consumer satisfaction strategy. This approach has several advantages. First, the costs of instrument development, analysis, and reporting can be shared among several providers. Second, reporting can compare each provider to the others. While comparisons will be made across a relatively small group, this approach is more valuable than the single-facility approach. This model is one that could be adopted by membership organizations of long-term care providers, managed care organizations, or others.

CONCLUSION

The steps to be taken and the decisions to be made regarding obtaining consumer input are many and varied. These questions include the following:

1. *How will you use the information? For negotiating managed care contracts? Improving service? Examining the effects of a new program or service?* Being clear about the goals of your work is the first important step. Outside evaluators are perceived as being unbiased, and so the results of their work may be more meaningful to managed care organizations or consumers making a choice to purchase your services. An American Association of Retired Persons (AARP) publication on selecting managed care plans warns consumers, "HMOs will report only the best results from a survey, not all the findings. The best type of surveys are those conducted by an uninvolved organization that uses a standard set of questions" (American Association of Retired Persons, 1996, 11). On the other hand, to work on an organizational plan for service improvement, an internal exploration using small-scale approaches may be all that is necessary.

2. *How much money do you have to spend, or how does the priority of collecting satisfaction information compare with other competing demands?* Consumer satisfaction as a high priority might dictate a large-scale approach, while a lower priority might dictate a

smaller-scale approach. Documenting the satisfaction of your consumers may result in tradeoffs among providing more services or raises for your employees. If you want a large-scale approach while using limited funds, where can you seek volunteer assistance, collaborators to share the cost, or other methods for funding your work?

3. *What is your client population like?* The characteristics of your population may often dictate the most appropriate approach to hearing their voices. Questions of frailty, literacy, telephone access, and cognitive abilities should all be considered when choosing the method for obtaining consumer input. What will your clients happily and easily do to make their voices heard?

4. *What should you ask your clients?* While we recommend a qualitative approach as a beginning point, many useful existing instruments may also be appropriate. If you perceive your organization as being similar to many others, without unique services or clientele, existing instruments have several advantages. On the other hand, if you survey your clients on issues that are not important to them, it is unlikely that you will be able to make meaningful service improvements or examine the effects of special services or service approaches.

5. *When is the right time?* Many organizations survey their clients every year, while others continuously collect satisfaction information. For example, some nursing homes mail surveys to each of their short-stay residents 2 weeks after they are discharged. To some extent, timing is dictated by the needs of the organization. Every-other-year might be often enough, particularly if cost is a concern. On the other hand, up- to-date input can provide insights to growing problems before they can become full blown. Needless to say, once is not enough. Organizations change, often drastically, and consumer satisfaction information collected 10 years ago probably has little relevance to your organization today. This year's answers may dictate a small-scale approach, while next year a large-scale approach seems called for. The trap of "we've always done this" is alluring, particularly where you can already chart changes in client satisfaction over time. But starting each consumer satisfaction project by re-examining your goals, your priorities, and

the options available to you, may move you in some new and exciting directions for gathering input from your consumers. Another benefit of regular surveys is their ability to convey the message to consumers that you consider their input important. Consider the Hawthorne effect, named after an experiment at the Hawthorne Electric Plant, in which different lighting conditions had no effect on employee productivity. Researchers found that the groups of employees participating in the study appreciated the attention so much that they maintained high productivity no matter what the condition. Asking consumers in your organization how they feel about their services is yet another way of letting them know that they are important to you.

As evidenced by the questions from the list above, deciding upon a strategy for a consumer satisfaction assessment is a process involving a number of choices and constraints. The following chapters provide some examples of how different organizations have designed consumer satisfaction approaches.

Part II

Approaches to Measuring Consumer Satisfaction

Chapter **5**

Measuring Consumer Satisfaction with In-Home Care

INTRODUCTION

In response to criticisms that our system of long-term care was biased toward the provision of care in a nursing home setting, there has been a dramatic expansion of inhome services. This transformation has occurred steadily over the past two decades, primarily through the Medicaid and Medicare programs, and through additional dollars allocated at the state level. The use of Medicaid for noninstitutional long-term care services has been a major catalyst to the home care movement. In 1982, 1.2% of the long-term care Medicaid expenditures were allocated to home care. By 1987, home care expenditures had risen to almost 10% of the total. Over the next decade, the growth continued with an increase to 13.4% in 1990, 16% in 1993, and 20.7% in 1996, accounting for over $10 billion in program expenditures. This expansion has occurred in three components of Medicaid, personal care services, home- and community-based waiver services, and home health care.

Growth has occurred in the Medicare home health program as well, rising from $2.5 billion in 1987 to over $12 billion in 1996, and estimated to approach $20 billion in 1998. Medicare has risen, in part, because of rule changes that expanded the number of providers, due to an expansion of home health benefits, and the implementation of the hospital prospective payment system.

Although the expansion of inhome care has been praised for providing more options for people with disability, it has also been accompanied by growing concern about the quality of care. Home care recipients often experience substantial levels of physical or cognitive limitations; they are, in many cases, alone and have contact with solely the care provider, and the service workers are typically poorly paid and minimally trained. Efforts to ensure the quality of inhome care encompass a range of approaches. However, a key element of any quality strategy is creating mechanisms to assess consumer satisfaction. This chapter will describe a series of approaches to collect data from consumers, including specific techniques and tools used.

HOMECARE DEFINED

Homecare is not a new phenomenon. The first formal home care agency in the U.S. was established in the 1880s (Phillips, 1989). The bulk of personal care and assistance for people with disabilities has always been provided at home and often by informal care givers. Despite this rich history, defining homecare has become a much more complicated task over the past decade or so, as the range of available services has broadened to include an array of medical and nonmedical services. Homecare can be divided into three major categories:

- *Environmental assistance* includes the key services typically available in a hotel setting, such as housekeeping, shopping, and laundry.
- *Personal care* assistance provides help with basic activities of daily living, such as bathing and dressing, assistance with instrumental activities, such as meal preparation; and other supportive services such monitoring.
- *Health-related care* includes various nursing and health services, such as administering medication; catheter and ostomy care; skin

care; and rehabilitation services. Health-monitoring and training in selfcare are also components of this category.

In addition to variation in the range of services included under the home-care definition, we find differences in the types of providers, the setting of service-provision, and the modes of financing and reimbursement. Each of these factors will influence our strategy for consumer assessment of satisfaction with inhome care.

HOME CARE CHALLENGES

To help guide our consumer satisfaction assessment strategy, we begin by examining the types of problems frequently reported for in-home care provision. An understanding of these issues will help as we develop outcomes, measures, and data-collection strategies for in-home care.

The range of services and providers does affect the nature of problems faced. For the personal care–type services, our experience, which comes from a range of research and demonstration programs and with state home and community-based care programs, suggests a common set of problems facing most home care programs. Typical home care challenges include: worker no-shows; failure to perform duties; lack of respect by worker; poor knowledge of health and skills tasks; inappropriate match of service recipient and worker; theft; and rough or abusive care, both physical and verbal. Because of the personal nature of in-home services, the relationship between worker and consumer is critical to quality. Although worker expertise is important, our research indicates it is not a substitute for limitations in the personal treatment of service recipients (Woodruff & Applebaum, 1996).

Skilled home health service provision must also balance the provision of technically sound care with the consumer's desire to be treated as an individual. Most of the home health concerns have focused on costs of care, fraud and abuse, and clinical outcomes. Several initiatives, such as the National League of Nursing Pulse study, have examined the consumer's view of health care.

APPROACHES TO ASSESSING CONSUMER SATISFACTION

As discussed in chapters 3 and 4, there are a number of ways to assess the consumer's satisfaction with the home care services received. Agency and researcher efforts described earlier include individual interviews completed in-person or by telephone; mailed surveys; consumer logs or diaries; focus groups; in-depth interviews or case studies; professional observations; interviews with family members or other care givers; and tracking consumer outcomes or complaints.

Before an agency actually begins to collect data from consumers, it is our recommendation that the agency develop an overall strategy for the consumer data collection effort. All data collection has costs to both the agency and researcher, and the consumer and their family. Although hearing the voice of the consumer is critical to quality care, delivering quality services remains the number one goal of the provider agency. The consumer data collection strategy must provide the minimal amount of data on which to make good decisions necessary to improve quality. Too much data collection means that services are sacrificed, while too little results in limited information on which to make critical decisions.

Developing a strategy for data collection requires that an organization look at a range of issues including agency size and budget; type of clients served, the customer groups served, including their requirements and expectations; level of internal expertise; industry norms; and level of commitment to quality improvement.

Data collection is expensive, and it is essential for organizations to self-assess on these issues in order to develop a strategy. Such an approach would include such components as assessing the resources available for consumer data collection, the type of information-processing system available, the need for outside consulting, client level of ability in responding to consumer satisfaction surveys, other assessments that consumers might be asked to complete; seasonal changes in agency practice that might influence consumers; indicators such as length of stay as an agency client who could effect data collection efforts, and other information that might be available to the organization.

Thus, any consumer data collection strategy is developed both in the context of an overall quality improvement effort and with the recognition of these factors. Once an approach has been identified, the next step is to detail the data collection activities within each specific area. As noted earlier, our recommended strategy involves a broad-based data collection approach that includes different types of consumer input. It is this strategy that combines both small-sample qualitative data collection, (i.e., focus groups), intermediate efforts (i.e., client logs or diaries), and larger-scale survey work, in order to provide the greatest insight into the consumer experience. The remainder of the chapter will discuss the application of these efforts within the home care arena.

Small-Scale Approaches

As identified in chapter 3, we recommend the use of small-scale approaches to gain insight into the consumer experience. Our work has used focus groups, indepth interviews, case studies, and consumer logs and diaries to collect data in this area.

Focus Groups

Focus groups described in chapter 3, are an excellent mechanism to gain detailed information about program operations or consumers' feelings on service access or provision. As a small and nonrandom sample, focus groups are not designed to provide a representative view of the services delivered, but rather as a technique to learn about what consumers think about service delivery. The focus group process is designed to use the interactions and experiences of consumers to learn more about service quality. Focus group topics are used to educate the provider on an area of concern or interest, in preparation for more extensive data collection activities.

As an example, a case management home care provider was considering using a clustered home maker–personal care service provision model in a senior housing complex. This delivery system option would provide services in shorter blocks of time throughout the entire day, rather than the traditional 2- or 4-hour blocks of time. It was hoped that the model would provide consumers with greater flexibility and thus improve the quality of services. Prior to implementation however, the agency wanted input from consumers, both on the concept and how the service option might be designed. Consumers expressed mixed feelings about the innovation. On one hand, they liked the idea that the worker could be available for them at multiple times during the day. On the other hand, they were concerned that their scheduled block of time might be too limited or that they would not have enough time with their worker.

Recognizing the potential issues, program staff attempted to design the service option to ensure an adequate block of time, and at the same time tried to educate consumers on how this service option could affect their care. The topics also alerted program planning and evaluation staff on what issues might affect consumer satisfaction. These could then be the subjects of more widespread data collection activities, such as consumer satisfaction surveys completed with a larger proportion of residents. Other focus group topics used in home care have included consumers' views on how they were treated when they applied for services, whether consumers should have more control over home care services and in-home workers, how the cost-sharing component of the home care program should be structured, and why consumers choose to terminate home care and enter an institutional residence.

Focus groups generally include 7 to 10 participants and a facilitator, and usually last between 60 and 90 minutes. Because of the small number of participants, it is not possible to have a random or representative sample of consumers, but you can attempt to pick consumers that represent different perspectives. In our work, we typically provide some type of renumeration to participants—either a small amount of funds ($15.00) to cover transportation costs, or a small gift. Home care consumers typically need assistance with travel, which we would routinely offer and provide.

In-Depth Interviews

In-depth interviews are also used to gain a better understanding of the consumer's view of service delivery. We use in-depth interviews in two ways. One is similar to the focus group goals, implemented to get more information about a specific idea or problem. The second is used as a specific quality and satisfaction assessment, to talk with consumers about the current services received.

The first approach is used when an agency is considering making modifications to a program or when an agency is concerned with program design and structure. For example, an agency, concerned that the initial assessment was too burdensome to the newly enrolled home care recipient, used an in-depth interview to discuss this question. In-depth interviews asked consumers about how they felt during the initial assessment, about their understanding as to why the comprehensive interview was important, and how this made them feel about the agency. Based on a series of in-depth interviews, the agency made two modifications: first, they did a better job of explaining why they needed to ask certain sensitive questions, and second, they decided that it was not necessary to complete every assessment question during that first meeting, as long as key items were ascertained.

The in-depth interviews to assess service quality and satisfaction have been used in some home care agencies as part of their quality assurance or improvement plan. In a quality improvement system that we designed for one state, consumers were chose in two ways to receive an in-depth interview; either at random from the agency caseload, or because they had reported some type of problem during the previous quarter. This mixed mode sampling strategy can be useful to agencies striving to hear the voices of consumers.

The in-depth interview process includes questions and probes abut the care received and the consumer's knowledge and feelings about their services. The in-depth quality improvement interviews include time for general discussion, specific questions about the services received and dialogue about the quality of life, their interactions with home care workers, and their thoughts on being an in-home care service recipient. The in-depth visits typically take between 75 and 90 minutes. Quality information about the performance of specific workers and agencies and a better understanding of what components of care are most integral to the consumer, are outcomes of this approach.

Findings from the in-depth interviews show that even with hesitant consumers such interviews can provide important insights into services. Data from interviews can be used to improve services from specific providers and help shape the array of services provided. The in-depth nature of the interviews provides a mechanism for consumers to share information and experiences that they might be reluctant or uncomfortable discussing with the provider. An example of specific feedback involved a consumer who after a one-hour interview hesitantly raised a complaint about her in-home worker, who she genuinely liked. "It really bothers me when Mary smokes," reported the consumer. Unfortunately for this consumer, who had emphysema, this was literally a life threatening complaint. In a second interview a consumer described a situation in which her personal care worker had stopped showing up to work when her television broke. In another interview a consumer who lived alone and had no informal assistance described a positive experience. Her personal care worker came to her home to provide assistance on her days off, because she knew that the consumer had no other service support.

Information from these types of interviews can be used by agencies to address both structural problems faced in the provision of services and specific problems or complaints. Although such interviews, which are completed on a small number of consumers do not represent a representative sample of problems, it does provide information about service delivery. Even if these problems are atypical, they need to be identified and addressed. These findings can also be used to inform larger scale data collection efforts as well.

Case Studies

Case studies are another technique used to help service providers hear from consumers. Such case studies involve an ongoing and in-depth look at a care situation. Case studies can involve interviews, observations, a review of records, or a combination of these activities. A case study could focus on a particular process (assessment, care planning, or consumer supervision of workers) or could include a more generic study of services. In a recent case study of the assessment and care planning process in a home care agency, members of our research team reviewed the assessment and care plan records for a sample of consumers, observed the assessment process, interviewed consumers, and interviewed care managers about the plan of care, in an effort to understand the strengths and weaknesses of the current approach. In another case study of home care clients, a member of our research team spent 3 months with six home care clients to learn from them what they thought was important to achieve quality of care. In this study the researcher would spend an hour or two each day with a home care consumer to watch and learn about quality. Study results highlighted the importance of consumer choice and autonomy in achieving quality of care (Woodruff & Applebaum, 1996).

The use of the case study technique is quite time-consuming and is less likely to be used by an organization, particularly with internal resources. However, it does lend itself very well to collaborative work. In many communities university students are looking for applied projects, and these types of opportunities could provide a model that would be mutually beneficial for agency and student. Its advantages are that such a technique provides a glimpse into the black box of quality care, that is often elusive using other types of approaches. Its disadvantages are that it is time consuming, expensive, and typically beyond the resources and expertise of an individual agency. The collaborative model is, however, one mechanism of addressing these limitations.

Consumer Diaries

Consumer diaries have been used in a number of research projects to elicit detailed information from study participants about areas such as health care utilization, service receipt, physical health and functioning, and consumer expenditures. Although this approach has not typically focused on consumer satisfaction, our work has shown that it lends itself well to this area of study. In this approach, consumers are provided with a diary and asked to record actions, reactions, observations, and thoughts or comments about the services received. There are a number of ways to implement this approach. Most studies provide some structure to the diary process by giving consumers specific areas to record, such as worker attendance, punctuality, use of replacement workers, and other descriptive items. Additionally, diaries have tried to include an assessment of services by asking consumers to record reactions to a series of quality dimensions, such as dignity and respect afforded to the consumer, knowledge of client conditions and service techniques, and willingness to meet consumer requests.

A Consumer Log

A consumer log—based on the concept of the Neilsen ratings—has been used as a mechanism for consumers to describe their service experience. In this effort, implemented in a recent demonstration, a randomly selected group of consumers was asked to participate as "Neilsen families". This concept, which was well known to consumers from their use in television, was readily accepted by respondents. The Neilsen home care rating approach was used for both personal care services and home delivered meals. Consumers selected were initially telephoned in order to describe the project, to assure that they were cognitively able to participate and determine potential interest. Those meeting the criteria were then visited in order to explain more about the expected responsibilities, to agree to participate, and to be trained on the log forms and process.

One week during each quarter consumers would receive logs in the mail to be completed and returned in an already stamped and addressed envelope. The log included both the opportunity to respond to specific questions and use the open-ended space for additional comments. For example, in the home delivered-meal category consumers were asked "Did the meal arrive on time?" "Was the driver respectful?" "Did the food taste good?" Consumers would answer this range of questions each day of the week. They would also record general observations within each of the areas and in a final summary section as well. A similar process was used for the personal care services.

The Neilsen approach had the advantage of the in-person interview in terms of initial training and orientation but was not as time-consuming or expensive. In general, once consumers had been visited in-person they took the "Neilsen Family" responsibility seriously. One example of this attitude took place during one of the test quarters. We had decided that it would be better to mail the log forms just a few days before the consumer was to complete his or her recording. In one quarter the forms were sent out late and had not arrived on the normal date for delivery. The participating agency received numerous phone calls from the Neilsen participants wanting to know why the logs had not yet arrived.

The logs or diary system do have some distinct advantages over the small- and large-scale data collection efforts. It allows the agency or researcher to sample a larger proportion of consumers, which provides more

confidence than the small scale-approaches. Such an approach also provides a great deal of insight into service delivery. Although not as gener-
alizable as the large scale survey efforts, it does provide more depth than
these efforts. For agencies with limited resources this approach provides
an opportunity to collect high-quality data from consumers at a lower cost
than would be possible with continual in-person techniques.

Electronic Communication

Electronic communication is another method now being used to dialogue
with consumers. This approach has been used in two major ways in previous work. In a Wisconsin study consumers are linked together to share
experiences about illness, services and treatment. In this case women at
home being treated for breast cancer have the opportunity to talk to other
women about both factual and emotional-care issues. A second approach
is for the provider to have electronic mail interactions with consumers.
Again, this could involve responses to specific questions from the provider,
an open chat or complaint line to the provider, or simply a mechanism to
encourage a dialogue or questions from consumers. The advantages of such
an approach is that it can be done a relatively low cost while providing the
opportunity to gain insights into service delivery. Access to technology and
the associated costs may mean that many older consumers would not be
able to participate in such an option. Such an option may become much
more viable in the future, as the use of the Internet becomes more like having the accessability of a telephone.

LARGE SCALE APPROACHES

Although the small-scale strategy provides richness in helping to understand how services are delivered and received, they can not be used as the
sole consumer assessment technique. The small-scale approaches are time
consuming and, because they are implemented with a small non-random
sample, an agency must be careful about overgeneralizing from the experience. For larger, more representative information, we rely on the social
survey—an approach well known to American culture. From election polls

to marketing telephone calls (especially during dinner) we have lots of experience with being surveyed. Three common forms of data collection—in-person, via telephone, and via mail—comprise the approaches typically used in consumer assessment. As discussed in chapter 4, issues such as cost of data collection, response rate, reliability and validity of information, and the types of information that can be asked are all affected by mode of data collection. In the remaining portion of this chapter we will examine efforts to assess consumer satisfaction using these three approaches.

Although each of the three modes have different strengths and weaknesses, there are some common principles of data collection that we believe are important, regardless of the technique. As noted in chapter 3, it is important to ask specific questions rather than the generic. For example, it is better to ask "Did your home care worker show up on time today?" rather than "How is the schedule for your in-home worker?" or even "Are you satisfied with your worker's attendance?" The generic satisfaction questions typically result in little respondent variation, or in practical terms, everyone reporting to be highly satisfied. Additionally, numerous other factors affect consumer responses including, such areas as question response categories, time of day and season, length of interview, type and style of interviewer or format of survey, decision rules on use of proxy respondents, and data collection process and respondents level of comfort in reporting attitudes about services. Although these factors influence data collection in each of the three modes, the effects of these differences may vary depending on the data collection approach. Potential differences will be examined as part of our review of home care assessment activities.

In-Person Interviews

In-person interviews are an excellent mode of data collection in assessing consumer satisfaction, particularly in working with individuals with chronic disabilities. The in-person interview typically relies on closed-ended questions and structured responses. As discussed earlier, we strongly recommend that questions be specific to the service area under investigation. For example, questions about homemaker or home health aide service would include such areas as my homemaker/home health aide leaves early, my homemaker/home health aide is rude to me, my homemaker/home health aide arrives late, and my homemaker/home health aide ignores what I tell her about how I like things done. Although a general satisfaction question can be asked, our experience suggests that most respondents report overall positive satisfaction, regardless of service quality. The specific questions do a far better job of identifying variation among consumers. Table 5.1 includes a review of select instruments used to assess satisfaction of home care recipients. Program differences, target population served, geographic location, cultural and ethnic differences, and numerous other factors will have an effect on question selection and appropriateness. Selection of survey question items will need to be made in the context of these factors.

The overview table includes examples from three instruments examining satisfaction with care management and in-home services. Although variation exists across the efforts, they share several common principles: ask specific questions, provide balanced response categories, collect data either in-person or over the telephone, and collect data across agencies to develop a comparative data base.

Use of the in-person interview for home care consumers has important strengths and weaknesses. In working with individuals with chronic disability, the in-person interview facilitates communication and enhances reliability of responses. Being in the home provides the interviewer with a better sense of the consumer and his or her family environment, which helps in determining response validity. Because a portion of the population receiving home care also experiences cognitive disability, the in-home assessment provides better information for determining if a respondent is capable of answering questions about services. The decision to use the actual consumer or a proxy to complete the survey is a continual issue in completing the assessment. An in-person assessment provides a more complete picture on which decision to make.

The in-person assessment also provides an opportunity to establish a rapport with a consumer, which may lead to higher quality data collection, as the consumer feels more comfortable with the data collection process.

The use of in-person home care assessment is not without limitations. Such interviews are costly. In 1997, $75 per interview was a typical cost estimate, with some data collection efforts considerably higher than that figure. Given travel and recording time, we typically budget no more than three in-home interviews in a day. Additionally, in many of our home care

Table 5.1 Measures of Consumer Satisfaction with In-Home Care

Instrument	Dimensions/Areas Assessed	Intended Population	Data-Collection Method
Home Care Satisfaction Measure (HCSM) (Geron et al., 1998)	Satisfaction with individual home care–, as well as overall home care services. 3–4 dimensions for each service are assessed. The dimensions for home maker and home health care are: competency, system adequacy, positive interpersonal, and negative interpersonal. For case management, they are: competency, service choice, positive interpersonal, and negative interpersonal. For homedelivered meals, they are: quality, system adequacy, and service dependability. For grocery service, they are: quality, system dependability, and service convenience.	Frail older adults who receive any of five home care services: home maker, home health aide, home delivered meals, grocery services, or case management	One subscale for each service; each contains 10–13 items. The HCSM contains 60 items in all. It is scored with a 5-point Likert response scale. Items and subscales are scored from 0–100. The time frame of the items is the present tense. In-person and self-administered versions are available.

Table 5.1 (continued)

Instrument	Dimensions/Areas Assessed	Intended Population	Data-Collection Method
Home Interview Tool Wisconsin Dept. of Health and Family Services (The Management Group, 1997)	Focuses on 3 dimensions of care: quality assurance, quality assessment, and customer satisfaction. Example questions include: I help decide which services I receive, My home care worker arrives on time, I can get hold of my case manager easily.	Frail older adults who receive care management, in-home services, or respite care	Instrument administered in-person. Scale includes 22 statements, 9 about case managers, 7 about in-home services, and 6 about substitute care. A 5-point Likert scale—"strongly disagree" to "strongly agree"—is used.
Ohio Quality Assurance Tool—Ohio's PASSPORT program	Asks a series of specific questions about service delivery such as—did the worker arrive on time—does the service worker smoke— does the client like and trust the service worker?	Frail older adults receiving home maker/personal care, home delivered meals, case managers, adult day care	Data collected in-person only: Yes/no response categories are the only choice. Time frame is the present tense.

studies consumers live in difficult-to-access or unsafe neighborhoods, making data collection more difficult and more expensive.

Although it has been argued that the in-home, in-person interview provides more reliable and valid data, there is another view point that suggests that consumers feel more comfortable giving results over the telephone or via the mail. Rather than providing a mechanism for consumers to feel more comfortable, this argument suggests that the in-person interview may be more inhibiting for the respondent. Unfortunately, studying the validity of research responses is difficult. What researchers can do is study different data collection approaches and compare results. Which results are correct however, is a different story. We do know that who collects the data, the circumstances of collection, how the survey is presented, and consumer comfort with the interview process will have a major effect on consumer responses. Decisions about the mode of data collection must consider these types of effects.

Telephone Interviewing

Telephone interviewing is perhaps the most common form of data collection in the survey research world. Because most U.S. households today have a telephone such a technique excludes very few (although it is the most vulnerable people in our society that would be most likely to be excluded). Telephone interviews have the advantage of being less expensive. We estimate completion costs at about 40% to 45% of the in-person interview. As noted previously, some researchers believe that the telephone provides for more freedom on the part of the respondent to provide valid answers.

Interviewing individuals with chronic physical and cognitive disabilities via the phone is not without considerable challenge. In addition to physical barriers to communicating over the telephone, there are issues about whether the respondent is capable and competent to complete the telephone assessment and whether the consumer is alone and free to respond without constraint from a formal or informal provider. Although we typically use a short battery of mental status questions to ascertain respondent ability, such an assessment over the telephone is difficult, and thus potential respondents might be screened in or out inappropriately. The telephone survey does not provide the interviewer with information about the situation surrounding the interview. Is the respondent alone or in a secure position to be interviewed? Although it is possible to ask questions about the social and physical environment, it is more difficult for the interviewer to exercise control over the interview situation over the telephone.

Although the final decision about the mode of data collection will depend both on the type of questions to be asked and the target population to be interviewed, expert opinion on the optimum mode of data collection is mixed. In some of our recent work we have compared the results of telephone assessment with in-person interviews for home care recipients (McGrew & Quinn, 1997). Results showed that while some differences existed on assessment questions, in general, the telephone assessment generated reliable data. Recent work has also identified the reliability of telephone consumer satisfaction survey techniques (Geron, 1996). Testing consumer satisfaction instruments on different target populations in different geographic locations, recent studies have been able to identify a series of measures that we believe will work for both practice and research objectives (Geron, 1996). This work uses many of the principles that we have discussed throughout the book. Ask specific questions that are simple, meaningful, and direct. The items were developed by using focus groups of consumers and providers to identify areas of service that are important. Questions were then tested and then statistically validated.

Based on these experiences, we believe that assessing satisfaction via the telephone is an effective approach for agencies. Although we believe that any data collection strategy should include an in-person validation component for an ongoing quality improvement effort, telephone data can provide reliable, valid, and less costly information about service quality and satisfaction.

Mail Surveys

Mail Surveys common in consumer marketing efforts, has been a typical strategy used by many home care agencies. The major advantages of such an approach are that they are relatively easy to implement, are nonintrusive to respondents, they provide anonymity to consumers, and they are inexpensive.

The disadvantage of this approach for assessing consumer satisfaction with in-home care is that, in most agencies, this approach has never worked. As we have travel around the country giving workshops on this topic we often ask agencies what technique they use to assess consumer satisfaction with services. Typically, 90% or more of the agencies in attendance have or are currently using a mailed satisfaction survey for their home care consumers. However, when asked how well they work the universal response is that everyone always reports high levels of satisfaction. "Either we are better then we think we are, or this doesn't work." In addition to little variability in response patterns, mailed surveys to consumers usually have low response rates, which typically result in a nonrandom or a biased sample of responders. This essentially means that the advantage of the mailed survey, which is to generate a random sample of consumers, is limited by a high and differing response rate.

Although mailed surveys have not realized a significant amount of success, they can be a useful component of an overall strategy. Again, our lessons for asking specific questions are reinforced with this approach. We find that a short battery of specific, time-focused, and direct question can work via the mail. Consumers need to be made aware of the importance of the effort, that their opinion counts, that the survey is quick to complete, and that the survey is easy to complete and can be returned in an addressed and postage-metered envelope. Again, we like to include a validation component in our overall strategy, such that the mailed survey response can be validated on a sample of consumers. If consumer responses are reliable then this provides evidence to suggest that the technique can be used effectively.

Suggestion Boxes

Suggestion Boxes are a variant of the mailed survey. Used in restaurants, libraries, and retail stores, this technique provides a mechanism for consumers to make comments or register complaints about the service or product delivered. The advantage of such an approach is that it is inexpensive and it provides consumers with a direct opportunity to report on an issue of concern. The disadvantage is that it is nonrepresentative and thus difficult to assess the nature and scope of the comment or complaint. Also, any time you provide consumers with an opportunity to comment it is important that the provider have a mechanism for responding to such comments. Thus, a comment or complaint box that gets ignored may be worse than not having a mechanism at all. Although perhaps a bit more relevant for residential long-term care settings, adult day care, outpatient health care, and other such locations could utilize such an approach.

CONCLUSION

In this chapter, we have highlighted the numerous strategies available to home care providers interested in hearing the voices of consumers. It is imperative that the specific data collection efforts be part of an overall data collection and quality strategy. This strategy should include amount of resources for the data effort, frequency of collection, mode of collection, the development of benchmarks, and a linkage and integration with an overall quality approach for the organization.

Chapter 6

Resident Satisfaction In Nursing Homes and Assisted Living

The nursing home industry is currently facing immense challenges. The growth of home-care, alternative care settings such as assisted living, and changes from retrospective to prospective reimbursement, have combined to change the way we think about nursing homes and the care they provide. Increasingly, those who need labor-intensive, sophisticated, 24-hour care, rather than custodial care, use nursing homes. Medicare, which pays for a nursing home stay after hospitalization, has increased the proportion of their budget spent on skilled nursing facility care from 1.2% in 1980 to 5.2% in 1995. In 1996, this amounted to just over $10 billion dollars (U.S. General Accounting Office, 1996; U.S. House of Representatives, 1997).

Medicaid, the largest public sector payer for nursing home care, spent $33 billion in 1997 (Burwell, 1998). Such high expenditures draw a considerable amount of attention from the public and elected officials. In response to concerns about quality of care, the Omnibus Budget Reconciliation Act of 1987 implemented many nursing home reforms. From the consumer's point of view, one of the most important reforms was the inclusion of interviews with residents as a component of the Medicaid/Medicare certification survey process. In this respect, the government has taken an important step in integrating consumer input into an overall assessment of facility quality.

While nursing homes have increased their take of the federal health care dollar they have also been serving a changing clientele. As Diagnostic Related Groups (DRGs) have resulted in shorter hospital stays, the nursing home is seeing increasingly more disabled short-stay patients, thus requiring treatments that are more sophisticated. For a segment of residents, the nursing home has come to resemble a hospital of an earlier era. Its use now is often as a transition from hospital to home. For example, in 1994 79% of nursing home residents with Medicare had stays of 40 days or less; 92% stayed for less than 80 days. (Komisar, Lambrew, & Feder, 1996).

Assisted living has increasingly become an alternative to nursing home care. Tremendous growth has occurred in assisted living care, as consumers express an interest in this more residential alternative to institutional long-term care. The shift to serving nursing home residents for a shorter time also has given a boost to the more residential assisted-living option. Assisted living properties generally provide less medically oriented care to residents who are not, generally, as impaired as those in nursing homes. A recent national study, found that assisted living residents, on average, needed assistance with 1.3 activities of daily living (ADLs) (Kramer, 1998), compared to needing assistance with 4.0 ADL limitations in nursing homes (Cowles, 1995). Since the 1980s, the assisted living industry has grown rapidly. By 1996, assisted living accounted for over one-half of all senior housing being constructed in the U.S. (Murer, 1997).

The philosophy of assisted living is also different from that of most nursing homes. The assisted living philosophy, as defined by the Assisted Living Federation of America includes the following goals:

- offering cost-effective, quality, personalized care
- fostering independence for each resident
- treating each resident with dignity and respect
- promoting each resident's individuality
- allowing each resident choice of care and lifestyle
- protecting each resident's right to privacy
- nurturing the spirit of each resident
- involving the family and friends, as appropriate, in care planning and implementation
- providing a safe, residential environment
- making the assisted living residence a valuable community asset

Because the philosophy of assisted living is very consumer-focused, the assessment of consumer satisfaction in the assisted living setting should be an integral part of most assisted living operations. Accordingly, the Assisted Living Quality Coalition (1998) recommended that the first task of any national quality organization for the assisted living industry should be the development and validation of consumer satisfaction measures (along with clinical and functional outcome measures). Clearly, performance-assessment in these areas is perceived to be integral to the quality of the industry.

NURSING HOME– AND ASSISTED LIVING CHALLENGES

As nursing homes have begun to serve a different population, strategies for assessing quality have also shifted. Donabedian's (1980) model of structure, process, and outcomes has long guided the assessment of health care quality. Historically, nursing home quality assurance mechanisms have always focused on organizational structure. Safe buildings, licensed staff, appropriate resident staff ratios, and licensed facilities were thought to be enough to ensure quality care. Later efforts to improve quality encompassed the process of care provision. A focus on care planning, provision of appropriate services, and increased attention to resident rights are all a part of the process by which care is delivered. As managed care plays an increased role in Medicare, quality assurance mechanisms move toward an increased emphasis on outcomes. What are the results of the care we provide? Managed care companies are particularly interested in how different treatments and practices produce different outcomes, with a particular emphasis on minimizing costs while maximizing positive outcomes. The current challenge is to determine the outcome measures appropriate for nursing home residents. Chronic illnesses do not easily lend themselves to expectations for recovery or dramatic improvements in functioning. What is clear, however, is that consumer satisfaction is one part of the outcomes for examination. A committee within the Institute of Medicine Division of Health Care Services suggested that health-related quality of life and satisfaction with care be given special research attention over the next 10 years (Feasley, 1999).

The assisted living industry, unlike nursing homes, has had only a limited focus on structure and process domains. The current state of the industry finds wide variation across and within states on the type of facilities and services offered by organizations calling themselves "assisted living." Well defined elements of organizational structure and the processes for delivery of care are currently being proposed and debated, as more states license assisted living as a special category of residential service delivery.

Another challenge for residential care settings is assessing satisfaction with the technical aspects of care. Consumers may be unable to recognize technically inadequate care and they may be similarly reluctant to criticize the facility in which they live. While firing an individual home maker might be only minimally disruptive, changing one's residence is much more difficult. Consequently, older residents of nursing homes (and probably of assisted living facilities) often minimize any discontent they feel with comments such as, "They have a lot of us to bathe. It's not their fault I can't have a bath in the morning"(Straker, 1993). Uman and Urman (1997) report that a large proportion of residents report satisfaction with substandard care in some areas. For example, 67% of residents who required toileting assistance were satisfied with toileting help, although they were only rarely taken to the bathroom. This leads to one of the most common problems faced in the assessment of consumer satisfaction: lack of variation. Everyone reports being satisfied, so distinctions between facilities or within domains in the same facility are impossible to make. A focus on objective rather than subjective questions can help to eliminate this problem. For example, asking residents if their meals are served at the right temperature, with hot foods kept hot and cold foods kept cold, may elicit very different responses than asking how satisfied they are with the food.

APPROACHES TO ASSESSING CONSUMER SATISFACTION

As is the case for all health and long-term care providers, residential care settings need to develop an overall strategy for examining consumer satisfaction. Such a plan recognizes that different approaches may be used from year to year in the context of an overall strategic design. Plan development is dependent on a series of factors, including facility expertise, resource availability, information requirements, and previous efforts and experience. A beginning strategy might be to conduct focus groups and individual interviews from which a quantitative questionnaire could be developed for use the next year. Existing quantitative instruments might be supplemented by focus groups directed to topics that were of particular interest to the facility. As discussed earlier, the development of a consumer satisfaction strategy is done within a series of constraints on time, expertise, and budget.

DIMENSIONS OF SATISFACTION IN NURSING HOMES AND ASSISTED LIVING

The measurement of satisfaction with nursing home care and assisted living care differs from satisfaction with home services and medical care, because these organizations provide not just care, but a total living environment. Consumer satisfaction dimensions for nursing homes encompass nursing and medical services, as well as services such as meals, laundry, housekeeping, and activities. For assisted living, additional emphasis might be placed on the dimensions of choice, privacy, or individualized care, which reflects the philosophy of the assisted living industry.

As previously noted, examining the dimension of satisfaction most salient to your customers is likely to yield the most information for improving quality. The difficulty with this approach, however, is that nursing homes have multiple customers. As noted in chapter 3, families and residents differ in the areas they consider most important to their satisfaction. Managed care companies and individuals may have very different viewpoints regarding which dimensions of care are most critical for resident satisfaction. As shown in Table 6.1 some commonly included dimensions of satisfaction include:

- physician services—expertise, communication, availability
- nursing services—expertise, communication, availability
- aides—communication/respect/caring style
- housekeeping—cleanliness, overall hygiene
- meals—temperature, taste, variety
- environment—safety, attractiveness

Table 6.1 Measures of Satisfaction with Nursing Home Care

Instrument	Dimensions/Areas Assessed	Intended Population	Data-Collection Method
Resident Satisfaction Interview (RSI) (Simmons et al., 1997)	Help and assistance, communication with staff, autonomy and choice, companionship, food and environment, safety and security	Residents; successfully used, with a large proportion of cognitively impaired residents	Face-to-face interviews: 42 items; 3-pt. response scale—"yes", "no", "sometimes"
Satisfaction Assessment Questionnaires (SAQs); (American Health Care Association, 1996)	Facility setting, staff-education, relationships, professionalism. (Other dimensions dependent on customer group.)	Separate SAQ for 3 different customer groups: (1) long-term care, (2) subacute care (3) assisted living	Self-administered survey: no. of items varies by customer group
Nursing Home Resident Satisfaction Scale (NHRSS) (Zinn et al., 1993)	Physician services, nursing services, other services (meals, room, privacy, schedule)	Nursing home residents; (used successfully with cognitively impaired)	Face-to-face interviews: 11 items scored along with 4-pt. Likert scale, from "not so good" to "very good"
Nursing Home Service Quality Inventory (NHSQI) (Davis et al., 1997)	Staff and environmental responsiveness, dependability and trust, personal control, food-related services and resources	Nursing home residents prescreened by informants	Face-to-face interviews: 32 items assessing perceptions, refined from a 52-item survey; 7-item Likert responses, ranging from "very poor" to "excellent" and "very dissatisfied"

Table 6.1 *(continued)*

Instrument	Dimensions/Areas Assessed	Intended Population	Data-Collection Method
Customer Satisfaction Instrument (Kleinsorge & Koenig, 1991)	nurses/aides, administration, staff empathy, food, housekeeping, home issues	Residents, family and concerned friends	Self-administered survey: 32 items, 5-pt. Likert responses, ranging from "strongly agree" to "strongly disagree"
Satisfaction of Residents and Families in Long-term Care (Norton et al., 1996)	Living environment, laundry, food, activities, staff, autonomy, dignity	Residents and families. (Used successfully with cognitively impaired.)	Face-to-face interviews: responses use 1–5 Chernoff faces or 3–rung ladders
Resident and Family Satisfaction Questionnaires (Ohio Health Care Association)	Living environment, health care, independence, food and dining, emotional support, visitors	Residents and families	Self-administered survey: Facilities self-administered. 21 items with 4-pt. Likert response categories, ranging from "very satisfied" to "very dissatisfied", or "definitely yes" to "definitely no"

The applicability of these dimensions to your facility depends on what areas you are most interested in, what areas you are strategically trying to improve, or what your residents and families have discussed as important. Figure 6.1 compares seven currently used questionnaires on the dimensions of satisfaction. Although there are several common domains as noted above, each instrument differs from the others, suggesting a lack of consensus on the most important dimensions of satisfaction in nursing facility care.

Satisfaction questionnaires, which include the same domains, may ask very different questions about them. For example, in a review of instruments assessing resident control in institutional settings, all instruments included the domain of food and dining. Different instruments, however, addressed meal schedules, resident input into meal planning and scheduling, entrée choices, dining room seating choices, dining partners, and the décor and furnishings of the dining room. As mentioned previously, items that assess overall subjective satisfaction with a particular domain may not be specific enough to actually be useful in improving services. Consider the question, "How satisfied are you with the meals and dining here?" Suppose you receive a number of dissatisfied responses. What is it you will work to change? Food choices? Recipes? Dining room décor? Seat assignments or chairs? Food temperature? Waiting in line for meals? While you know that something is unsatisfactory, you've learned little that will assist in solving the problem. Another problem with broad questions is that the vast majority of respondents often answer positively to these types of questions. On the other hand, you have now learned about an area that might be important to follow up on with a different approach. Focus groups or individual interviews could delve into the dining experience to get at specific problems. Overall subjective questions can be useful for pointing you in the direction of problem areas; specific subjective questions give you information about what kinds of changes actually need to be made.

AN OVERVIEW OF EXISTING INSTRUMENTS

The selection or development of a structured quantitative instrument is often a difficult and sometimes paralyzing decision for an organization. The reasons for using existing instruments include the ability to compare your facility with others or with published benchmarks, established reliability and validity, and reduce the time and expertise needed for measure development. Comparisons over time and with other facilities can only be made when questions are asked the same way each time. Even if you have decided to develop a measure of your own, existing measures often provide a starting point for development. Ideas about how questionnaires should be organized, the areas to be included, appropriate answer formats, and overall style can be identified from a careful examination of existing instruments. The information provided in the following sections will assist in our evaluation of questionnaires in this chapter and should also prove helpful to you in evaluating satisfaction tools that you may locate on your own.

There are several important areas that are critical to good instrument development. Whether evaluating existing instruments or designing your own, particular attention should be given to (1) overall organization, (2) areas covered, (3) reading level and question wording, and (4) response categories.

Overall Organization

In general, questionnaires and surveys should be designed to engage participants in the process. Questionnaires usually move from simple questions to more complex. Requiring complex or difficult judgments to be made early on may discourage some participants from completing the interview or survey. In addition, clear instructions at the beginning and transition paragraphs between sections on different topics help participants understand what is expected from them and help in shifting their thinking from one topic to the next. Herzog and Rodgers (1992) suggest that less important questions be placed at the end, and that long sequences of questions should be broken up by changes in topic areas or physical activities. Look at the organization of existing instruments with an eye to their organization. If you add questions or reorganize existing instruments, previous measures of reliability and validity no longer hold, thus adapting an instrument removes the advantage of previously established reliability and validity. On the other hand, you may have a questionnaire that better meets your needs. In addition, if the mode or methods of administration change, then reliability may change as well. For example, a written survey previously handed out by a physician in the office might get very different results if mailed or administered during an interview.

Reading Level and Question Wording

As discussed in chapter 4, interviews and surveys may be intimidating to some respondents. A good questionnaire will be comprised of brief, clear statements or questions. Words should be chosen carefully so that there is no doubt as to their meaning. Clarity of meaning is one of the results of pretesting; when conducting interviews it becomes very clear which items are unclear in their meaning or may have several different interpretations. Many computer word processing programs have features that will allow you to check the reading level of items; a reading level of 8th grade or below is recommended.

It is also crucial to ask the questions that you mean to ask. Consider the difference between "The nurse aides usually treat me with respect" and "The nurse aides treat me with enough respect". The first item is assessing frequency of respectful treatment, while the second item addresses the degree of respect being given. One may be more appropriate or more important to your residents than another. Is consistency of treatment most important? Is the quality or type of treatment most important? This example leads to another problem area: "double-barreled" questions. The double-barreled question is one that addresses two areas. The item "The nurses usually treat me with enough respect" examines both frequency of treatment and the quality of the treatment. When a resident disagrees, which are they disagreeing with? Does a poor result on this question mean that you should work with your aides to be consistent in their treatment, or should you work on strategies for increasing their respect toward residents?

Response Categories

Questionnaires usually have structured response categories with a range of responses such as "strongly agree", "agree", "neither agree nor disagree", "disagree", "strongly disagree"; "yes" or "no"; or "excellent", "good", "fair", or "poor". The number and type of responses can have a dramatic impact on your survey results. For example, "strongly disagree" has an exact counterpart in "strongly agree", but where is the direct counterpoint to excellent? Zimmerman, et al (1996) point out that "there is no balanced contra response to excellent, and as a result, questions are often structured with more positive responses than potentially negative responses". A question that uses the response categories "excellent", "very good", "good", "fair", and "poor" has four out of five response categories that have some positive weight. Given that older adults are generally more likely to express satisfaction, the importance of not weighting questions with positive response categories is clear. "Yes" or "no" questions have generally been avoided in research, but for adults with mild cognitive impairments they have been used successfully.

EXAMPLES OF INSTRUMENTS

The Ohio Health Care Association (OHCA) provides a consumer satisfaction survey process to their member facilities. OHCA mails the surveys, tabulates results, and provides reports on how each facility compares with all the others surveyed at the same time. In addition, they will provide comparisons on an individual facility's scores over time to examine areas of change. The 21-item survey instrument uses broad questions and is designed to help facilities zero- in on areas for further examination. They suggest following up in problem areas with additional surveys of very specific questions, focus groups, interviews, or other activities to determine exactly what issues are problems. Questions such as "How satisfied are you with the food?" do not give administrators much information to plan improvements. They do, however, let administrators know that a discussion should be held with residents and families about the aspects of the food service that need to be improved.

The American Health Care Association (AHCA) has also developed a series of instruments available free of charge upon request. The instruments are provided for facilities to self-administer to different categories of residents and staff. They also market a system called "The Facilitator," which combines customer satisfaction data and Minimum Data Set 2.0 data to generate overall quality reports. Because the questionnaires are already designed and the software needed to generate reports is provided, facilities with little or no expertise in customer satisfaction can easily implement this survey strategy. The advantage of using instruments provided by an organization is that it provides ability to compare your facility with others. As more facilities participate, the database for comparisons grows. Some departments, such as food service, are always less satisfactory than others. A comparison of your food service with national or state averages may give you very different information than comparisons across departments. While your food service may be low in comparison to activities, it may actually be one of the most satisfying food service operations around. The series of AHCA instruments includes assisted living, subacute facilities for the mentally retarded, nursing homes, and families. This also allows you to compare across different levels of care in your own organization.

One instrument that has been well tested for use in nursing homes is The Nursing Home Resident Satisfaction Scale (Zinn, Lavizzo-Mourey, & Taylor 1993). This 14-item scale includes questions on physician services, nursing services, and other services, such as meals, rooms, and schedules. This instrument was tested with two groups of nursing home residents; even those with mild cognitive impairment as measured by the Mini-Mental Status Exam were able to understand and respond to the questionnaire items. The scale shows high reliability. One of the drawbacks of the instrument may be its heavy weighting on physician services. Four out of 10 questions on physician services is probably too many, given the role that physicians typically play in nursing facility care.

A second instrument that has also been well tested is known as the Nursing Home Satisfaction Scale. Developed in 1982, the Nursing Home Satisfaction Scale has 17 items designed to examine satisfaction with the environment and care givers (Kruzich, Clinton & Kelber, 1992). The items cover a variety of domains and include some factual questions about the facility, such as "At night you have a choice of going to bed when you want" and other more subjective items, such as "Life here is better than you expected when you first came here." Relationships between nursing home satisfaction and other organizational variables have been found, suggesting construct validity as well.

Norton, van Maris, Soberman, and Murray (1996) have extensively documented the development of an instrument tested in eight long-term care facilities in Canada. Called the Long-Term Care Resident Evaluation Survey, it has undergone testing and revision. Items cover seven domains:

living environment, laundry, food, activities, staff, autonomy, and dignity. One of the most distinguishing features of their instrument was its success in assessing care of the cognitively impaired residents. This may be due to their unique strategy of using faces and ladders with rungs to represent different resident responses.

Other researchers have also had success with interviewing cognitively impaired nursing home residents. Uman and Urman (1997) created a structured instrument from the results of qualitative interviews. Their approach consisted of asking residents what kinds of activities/practices were essential to quality, then compiling specific, observable behaviors related to quality into a questionnaire. Their approach has several advantages. First, it tells staff what practices are related to quality. Next, it relies on objective questions by asking residents if those specific practices actually occurred. This approach provides specific information that can easily be implemented into strategies for quality improvement. Finally, 79% of the nursing home residents were able to complete the interviews. Extensive reliability testing was used with a Screening Interview Schedule to identify only 15% of the nursing home residents who could not be interviewed.

USING CONSUMER SATISFACTION DATA IN YOUR NURSING HOME

To get your employees and staff on board for measuring consumer satisfaction, they need to feel confident about how the results will be used. The worker who says to a resident, "Now, don't say anything mean about me. We want housekeeping to do well" may cause the facility to miss important information about organizational performance that could improve care. Instead of using satisfaction results to reward or punish, such data need to be used for improvement. Rather than pitting your employees against each other, it would be more useful to compare data across facilities.

Problem areas can be turned into goals for improvement by workgroups of residents, frontline staff, and management. Strategies for reaching those goals can be developed to put consumer satisfaction at the forefront of day-to-day operations. Meister and Boyle (1996) suggest the following three steps for integrating consumer information into an overall quality improvement program: (1) disseminating results, (2) developing and implementing an action plan, and (3) reassessing consumer satisfaction. Results should be disseminated to those who responded, preferably through a meeting that would allow for discussion of topics beyond the questionnaire. In addition, staff should be informed of results so that departmental workgroups or committees could begin designing action strategies for improvement. Management should also be informed of the overall survey results, as well as the board of directors. All of these groups have different reasons for needing consumer satisfaction results.

Action plans can address areas of weakness and strength. Departments or issues that are highly successful can work with other departments or on other issues to share strategies for success. Workgroups, often used as part of a quality management strategy, can be brought together around single issues or to develop action plans for the facility as a whole. Regardless of their charge, they should be comprised of representatives from all levels and departments in the organization and focus on consensus building.

Reevaluating consumer satisfaction on a periodic basis also provides feedback for further quality improvements. New surveys can be compared to the old to chart progress. Progress and improvement provide information about the most successful action strategies. Declines or continued low scores in other areas produce additional information for new action plans, and new satisfaction initiatives. By utilizing your consumer satisfaction results in these ways, the information provides an important part of a quality maintenance and improvement program.

The only absolute wrong choice you can make in developing a strategy for nursing home or assisted living consumer assessment is to choose to do nothing. Accrediting bodies, such as Joint Commission on accreditation of Healthcare Organizations now require consumer satisfaction studies, and we anticipate that this trend will carry over to state and federal regulatory bodies in the future. Top facilities are also paying greater attention to consumer views and such improvement information could widen the quality gap across facilities. Most importantly, consumer information can improve both the quality of services and the quality of life for residents.

Chapter **7**

Measuring Consumer Satisfaction with Health Care

INTRODUCTION

Health care in the United States has undergone profound changes in the past three decades. New methods for financing and delivering care, new organizations for providing care, and a new array of settings where services are delivered have combined to fundamentally alter the health care landscape (Bodenheimer & Grumbach, 1995). One intriguing aspect of this revolution has been the 'discovery' of quality problems in health care and acknowledgment by providers of the importance of patient evaluations of care.

Until the 1970s, the only authoritative parties to a medical or mental health decision for most Americans were the patient, the provider and, at times, the patient's family. This was the outgrowth of a very "simple" but powerful model in which patients (consumers) paid only a fraction of the real cost of health care, health insurers received monthly premiums from consumers and contributions from organized payers of health care (especially employers, who contribute to the health care of their employees and the government); and the insurer paid the health care provider (physician, hospital, home care agency, nursing home or pharmacy) retrospectively or on a fee-for-service basis. Providers determined how much to charge for care and the insurers or payers simply paid the bills.

This system began to erode in the 1970s for a number of reasons: the increasing availability of medical technology and other advances in medicine; the growing number of older Americans and persons with disabilities in the population; and the persistent problems of medical malpractice. However, the rapidly rising costs of health care, fueled by all of these factors, had the central role in shaping the present system. The health care environment has experienced a revolution so complete that it bears almost no resemblance to the environment that prevailed just after World War II, nearly 60 years ago, and even in 1970, less than 30 years ago.

The most dramatic changes have been the rise of managed care and the shift from traditional fee-for-service payment toward prospective payment systems, including Medicare's Diagnostic Related Groups (DRG) system and capitation arrangements in managed care plans. Managed care has many definitions, but the core definition of managed care is a health care delivery system which integrates the previously separated system of delivery and financing. This is accomplished by contracting with physicians, hospitals, and other providers to offer a defined set of services to enrollees who meet agency-specified eligibility criteria, usually for a pre-specified or capitated monthly premium (Iglehart, 1992).

Originally developed in the 1920s, managed care has experienced explosive growth over the past two decades. Over 50 million people are currently enrolled in managed care organizations, approximately 20% of all Americans. Some estimate that 40%–50% of all U.S. citizens will receive care from managed care organizations within 5 years. The variety and number of managed care plans continues to grow. The clear trend is toward conventional insurance plans adopting cost containment measures associated with managed care plans. Preadmission certification, utilization review, and other managed care initiatives have been implemented by most conventional insurers, primarily to control inappropriate use of hospital inpatient care. Prospective payment and capitation has also accelerated the decrease in hospital utilization and the dramatic increase in use of ambulatory services in the last decade.

Another related change has been the corporate transformation of the U.S. health care industry. Increasingly, large corporations have integrated a previously decentralized hospital system, entered a variety of other health care businesses, and consolidated their control and ownership. Foremost has been the emergence of investor-owned hospital chains. A major component of this trend has been the horizontal and vertical integration of health care facilities into larger, more-centralized organizations. Several hundred for-profit and not-for-profit hospitals integrated horizontally into chains to obtain economies of scale and vertically to supply comprehensive services, ranging from health insurance to community-based outpatient care. This trend has been accompanied by an influx of a new class of administrators and the introduction of entrepreneurial and business values that often clash with the traditional health care values (McArthur & Moore, McArthur, 1997).

QUALITY OF HEALTH CARE

Under the traditional system, patients with health insurance had almost unlimited freedom to select a provider of their choice, but the physician had sovereignty over all clinical decisions. A patient's physician decided how much care a patient would receive, of what kind, and by which providers. The only restraints on providers were their oaths, ethics, and their wish to retain patient loyalty and fear of malpractice charges. Not surprisingly, the quality of care was also viewed as the health care providers' domain; accordingly, their assumptions about quality and how to assess it are reflected in past initiatives to define quality and set up mechanisms for assuring the quality of care.

In health care, quality is generally assessed by the three criteria proposed by Donabedian (1966): structure, process, and outcome. Structural criteria apply to the provider or program as a whole, including physical structures, equipment, record keeping, staffing, and administrative procedures (e.g., physician specialties in or ownership status of a hospital). Essentially, structural criteria refer to the programmatic elements considered necessary to provide adequate quality. Process criteria refer to the way procedures are handled between physicians and other health professionals and patients, and are designed to assess the adequacy of the procedures undertaken. In contrast to structural and process criteria, both of which deal with inputs, outcome criteria refer to the actual accomplishments of a program or the results received.

For providers, it was by and large presumed that health care had a positive impact on patients' health. After all, since the turn of the century, U.S. medicine led the world in identifying and reducing the risks of death and disease. Moreover, each year in the U.S. millions of people visited hospitals, physicians, and other care givers and received medical care of superb quality. Partly because the quality of care was considered indisputable, and partly because until recently there were no available means to either question or buttress these presumptions, structure and process criteria, rather than outcomes, were traditionally advanced as the core of health care quality assessment. Outcomes from the patients' perspective (i.e., satisfaction) or from the payers' perspective (i.e., efficiency or cost) were noticeably absent. The patients' views of the quality of care were not solicited since patients were not considered valid assessors of care quality.

This relative lack of attention on quality assessment in general, and the use of outcomes in particular, contrasts sharply with the many concerns now raised about quality. Since the breakdown of the traditional system of health care, due to resource limitations and emergence of concerns about patient care in the new era of managed care, there is growing recognition that the quality of health care cannot be assured and has not been sufficiently addressed. Not all patients' interactions with the health care system produce positive outcomes. An estimated 180,000 people die each year in the U.S. as a result of physician-caused injuries, and it has been estimated that 70% of these deaths are a result of errors and are therefore potentially preventible (Leape, 1994). In the past decade, interest in developing specific measures to define, assess, or assure quality has grown, and the focus is moving from process and structure to outcomes. One gauge of the intense interest in quality of care is a recent six-part series in *The New England Journal of Medicine* (Blumenthal, 1996). Other major health journals, such as *Health Affairs*, have also devoted recent issues to increasing consumer choice and information about health care quality (Iglehart, 1996; Edgman-Levitan & Cleary, 1996). Patients and payers are demanding data on outcomes in order to assess whether changes in the health care system have reduced quality.

Patient satisfaction assessment is an important part of this trend. Today's competitive health care environment has generated an unprecedented interest in assessing the quality of care, including a demand for consumer feedback on health plans, including satisfaction assessments. Health providers are increasingly having to justify what they do to compete with insurance companies for public and private dollars. The assessment of patient satisfaction is seen as an important tool in the strategy to be able to compete on the basis of quality and price. In selecting plans, consumers and the plan purchasers acting on their behalf want to know how enrollees assess their plans. Most health plans and health providers regularly survey their own customers to learn how to improve quality and market share and to comply with standards, such as Health Plan Employer Data In formation Set (HEDIS), established by the National Committee for Quality Assurance (NCQA) as a standard set of performance measures for plan to plan comparisons.

A REVIEW OF THE LITERATURE ON PATIENT SATISFACTION WITH HEALTH CARE

Measures of patient or consumer satisfaction with health care provide a unique source of information about the success of health care interventions, whether in the hospital, office, or community (Cleary & McNeil, 1988; Geigle & Jones, 1990). Patient satisfaction with care is also closely related to health status, as it provides information about the patient's utilization and evaluation of services provided. The use of measures that meet standard psychometric criteria of reliability and validity provide a more scientific basis on which to measure satisfaction with health care than simply asking clients, "How do you like the services you are receiving?"

A considerable body of health care research that has examined the use of consumers in the assessment of service quality involves patient satisfaction with physician or acute care (Hulka, Zyzanski, Cassel & Thompson, 1970, 1971; Ware, Snyder & Wright, 1976a, 1976b; Stamps & Finkelstein, 1981; Davies & Ware, 1988). In the past decade, researchers have explored patient satisfaction with nursing care (Lucas, Morris & Alexander, 1988; Hinshaw & Atwood, 1988; Eriksen, 1987); rehabilitation services (Davis & Hobbs, 1989); pharmacy services (MacKeigan & Larson, 1989); non-physician encounters in small hospitals (Guzman, Sliepcevich, Lacey, Vitello, Matten, Woehlke, & Wright, 1988) and other types of health care organizations, such as HMOs (Cryns, Nichols, Katz, & Calkins, 1989). Several extensive reviews of this literature have been completed (Lebow,

1974, 1983; Linn, 1975; Ware et al., 1976a; Locker & Dunt, 1978; Pascoe, 1983; Lochman, 1983; Cleary & McNeil, 1988; Yi, 1990; Aharony & Strasser, 1993).

Existing measures of patient satisfaction with medical care have been found to correlate with attitudes toward the community, satisfaction with life, values or expectations regarding medical services, health status, education, income, ethnicity, and geographic location, but many studies report contrary findings (Cleary & McNeil, 1988). Age has consistently been found to be related to satisfaction, with older patients reporting higher levels of satisfaction than do younger patients (Locker & Dunt, 1978; Linn, 1975). However, Geron (in press) found no differences among satisfaction responses for older adults' regarding home care services, suggesting age-affected decision-making diminishes among the elderly. Women also report higher satisfaction levels than men. Satisfaction measures have not been found to be consistently related to objective indicators or independent reports of patient quality (Davies & Ware, 1988; Gauthier, 1987). For example, Eriksen (1987) found negative correlations between subjective ratings of nursing care with objective assessments of care quality.

One distinction that is relevant when considering measures of patient satisfaction is the difference between objective ratings versus subjective reports (Davies & Ware, 1988). Client ratings represent the individual's subjective evaluation of care. This subjective assessment can be based on past experience and personal standards used in making the evaluation. Alternatively, objective reports represent events that did or did not occur. For example, an example of an objective report would be "Was the lunchtime meal served no later than 12:15 p.m.?" Reports are inherently more objective and can be confirmed by independent assessors, but have not been found to be highly correlated with a person's subjective assessment of the service under review (Davies & Ware, 1988; Roberts et al., 1983).

MEASURES OF PATIENT SATISFACTION

When considering a measure to assess patient satisfaction with health care, there is both good news and bad news to report. The good news is that there are a number of measures available for almost any particular service, and that some of these are well established, have been thoroughly tested for validity and reliability, and were designed for use with older adults. The bad news is that most of the existing measures possess a well known list of shortcomings. Most are service- or location-specific, that is, most involve the evaluation of specific services and cannot be used to make comparisons across programs. Most instruments lack the psychometric testing or standardization needed to allow reliable comparisons across health plans, population groups, or over time. Finally, most surveys use questions that are institution-specific or are designed to answer questions from the purchasers' or employers' point of view rather than the consumers'.

As with other types of satisfaction measures, measures of patient satisfaction can be single-item or multiple-item in length, global or multidimensional in design, geriatric or nongeriatric in focus. Below, we describe some of the most sophisticated efforts to assess patient satisfaction with care using standardized measures.

Single-Item Measures

Single item measures of patient satisfaction have been used for decades. Single item measures generally ask respondents to rate global feelings of satisfaction such as "Overall, how satisfied are you with the services you are receiving?" Among the research literature, a variety of single-item measures have been extensively studied (Andrews & Withey, 1976). Among the best of these is the Cantril ladder, a self anchoring scale of "0" to "10", on which "0" represents the worst possible life and "10" represents the best possible life. In our own research, we created a global satisfaction rating scale for various home care services as part of the research to develop the Home Care Satisfaction Measure (HCSM) (Geron, 1998). The basic scale was a 20cm visual analogue scale in the shape of a vertical thermometer with the end points clearly identified. Subjects were shown a thermometer for each service they received and asked to rate their overall satisfaction with that service. Respondents indicated their opinion by placing a mark on the thermometer. The distance to the mark from zero was measured in centimeters to the nearest millimeter and converted to a "0 to 100" scale.

Single-item or short multiple-item global measures have the advantage of ease of use and will obviously be less costly to administer than longer multiple-item measures assessing multiple dimensions of long-term care, although they are now generally discounted by researchers because the multidimensionality of long-term care services is now widely acknowledged. This point can not be stressed enough. In the area of acute care and in our own research in home care, research has established that long-term care is complex and multifaceted, even though the dimensionality has not been fully explained for each area or long-term care service. Single or multiple-item global measures of client satisfaction have an inherent weakness in that they factor in all relevant "weightings" of dimensions by respondents and do not allow the practitioner to assess what particular aspects of services are liked and disliked.

Multiple-Item Measures

Among multiple-item measures, there are several measures that are long established, well tested on a variety of populations, and relatively brief. Table 7.1 summarizes the characteristics of some of the established multiple-item measures of patient satisfaction with health care that have been developed. The following summary of three of the main instruments in use illustrates how these instruments are structured, the dimensions of satisfaction tapped, and the types and structure of questions that are included.

The Patient Satisfaction Questionnaire (PSQ), constructed by Ware and his associates (Ware and Snyder, 1975; Ware et al., 1976) is a carefully constructed measure of satisfaction with physician and medical services that addresses the following domains: availability of services, financing care, humaneness of doctors, quality of care, continuity of care, facilities, and general satisfaction. These scales are comprised of 2–4 items, and client responses are indicated on a 5-point Likert scale, ranging from "strongly agree" to "strongly disagree". Scale items are balanced in terms of positively and negatively worded items, to reduce acquiescent response bias (Ware, 1978). The PSQ has been widely used in the study of client satisfaction with health care (Guzman et al., 1988) and in validation of other scales.

The Client Satisfaction Questionnaire (CSQ) developed by Larsen, Attkisson, Hargreaves, and Nguyen (1979) is an 8-item instrument originally used to evaluate mental health services but was intended as a global

Table 7.1 Measures of Patient Satisfaction with Health Care

Instrument	Dimensions/Area Assessed	Time Frame of Assessment	Purposes/Intended Population	Data Collection Method
Client Satisfaction Questionnaire (CSQ) (Larsen et al., 1979)	Overall client/patient satisfaction	Present	Adults-consumer satisfaction with health and human service programs	Original version contained 18 items scored with a 4-point Likert response scale; revised version contains 8 items. Can be self-administered
Patient Satisfaction Scale (PSS) (LaMonica et al., 1986)	Technical-professional relationship Knowledge Trusting relationship Educational relationship	Present impression based on past experience	Outpatient (adult) satisfaction with nursing care	25 items item self-report scale; uses a 5-point Likert response scale
Patient Satisfaction Questionnaire (PSQ) (Ware et al., 1978)	Convenience of services Availability of services Financing care Humaneness of doctors Quality of care Facilities General satisfaction	Present (medical care received recently)	Health care patients	Original version contained 56 items (Form I) with a 5 point Likert response scale; revised 43 item version

Table 7.1 *(continued)*

Instrument	Dimensions/Area Assessed	Time Frame of Assessment	Purposes/ Intended Population	Data Collection Method
Older Patient Satisfaction Scale (OPSS) (Cryns et al., 1989)	Undifferentiated positive regard for HC providers; concern about quality of care; ease of access; complaints about waiting time; HMO is for routine care; appreciation of the treating physician, special care for serious problems; doctor informs about tests; good value for money; continuity of physician-provider access difficulties; availability of regular provider; general appreciation of the HMO	Current satisfaction based on HMO experiences	Older HMO patients 65+	60 item self-report instrument using a 5 point Likert response scale

measure of client satisfaction with human services, including health and medical care. Each of the items is rated on a 4-point Likert-type scale. In a study examining the correlation of the CSQ with service utilization and psychotherapy outcome (Attkisson & Zwick, 1982), the CSQ was correlated with greater symptom reduction and number of therapy sessions attended. No significant differences have been found when the CSQ has been used with different ethnic populations in a study of client satisfaction in two community mental health centers (Roberts & Attkisson, 1983). The CSQ has also been widely used (Heath et al., 1984). In a comparison of an 18-item version of the CSQ and the PSQ, Roberts, Pascoe and Attkisson (1983) found that the PSQ was significantly related to global or multidimensional measures of subjective well-being. They argue that satisfaction measures, such as the PSQ, that contain items about health care providers in general are more likely to tap components of subjective well-being, while satisfaction measures, such as the CSQ, that contain items referring specifically to services are more likely to assess service satisfaction.

The Older Patient Satisfaction Scale (OPSS) is a 60-item instrument constructed to measure older patient satisfaction with health care in HMOs. This measure, constructed by Cryns et al. (1989), was derived from consumer attitudes towards HMO services in a series of group interviews. From these group sessions, 11 content categories were identified in addition to one unclassified category: (1) physicians, (2) finances; appointments, (3) alternate providers, (4) changing doctors, (5) completeness of services, (6) convenience of the HMO, (7) personal health problems, (8) accessory programs, (9) atmosphere and feelings-general comments, (10) access and location, (11) preventive health care, (12) physical examination, and "unclassified". The OPSS correlates moderately well with the PSQ dimensions (.18 to .47), and CSQ (.40).

RECENT PRIVATE AND FEDERAL INITIATIVES

Recent public and private initiatives have moved the collection of consumer information into the forefront of quality improvement efforts in health care. We describe two of the largest efforts to date.

Consumer Assessments of Health Plans Study

In 1995, the Agency for Health Care Policy and Research (AHCPR), a federal agency operating under the Public Health Service, funded a new initiative called Consumer Assessments of Health Plans Study (CAHPS). The overall goal of CAHPS is to provide an integrated set of standardized survey questionnaires that can be used to collect and report meaningful and reliable information about the experiences of consumers enrolled in health plans. CAHPS is not a satisfaction measure, but collects information related to care quality that consumers would find helpful to know when considering a health plan, such as access to care, quality of care provided, and the communication skills of the providers and administrative staff. CAHPS is designed for use with all types of health insurance consumers, including Medicaid and Medicare beneficiaries, as well as the privately insured; and across the full range of health care delivery systems, from fee-for-service to managed care plans. It is also designed to capture information about special groups, including individuals with chronic conditions and disabilities, and families with children.

To carry out the CAHPS study, AHCPR awarded three 5-year cooperative agreements to consortia headed by RAND, Harvard University Medical School, and Research Triangle Institute. The CAHPS project has been divided into two major phases. During Phase I of its work, the three CAHPS grantees and Westat, a research consulting firm, have worked as a collaborative team to develop and test questionnaires that collect information on consumers' experience and assessments of health plans and services, develop and test different reporting formats for conveying this information to consumers, and design and implement an evaluation to improve CAHPS processes and products. In Phase II, a major objective was to understand how all the products—surveys, reporting products, implementation handbook—work in diverse, real-world settings. To obtain this information, the CAHPS grantees began working in early 1997 with five demonstration sites to implement the entire CAHPS Survey.

Together with the demonstration sites and early adopters, CAHPS grantees will conduct both process and outcome evaluations. The goal of the process evaluation is to learn where CAHPS processes and procedures succeed and fail when sponsors use them in real-world settings. The CAHPS team also will test some methodological questions in the demonstration sites, relating to mode effects (Does mail/telephone yield a higher response rate? Do responses vary systematically with one mode or the other, e.g., are telephone responses more positive?) and type of respondent (How do responses to the child health survey differ when completed by parent versus adolescent?). Starting in 1998, the CAHPS team will review all the lessons from the demonstration sites, early adopters, and other users. The CAHPs will then revise the products and procedures, disseminate the next versions of CAHPS products, and implement them in a second round of demonstration sites, budget permitting.

The Health Plan Employer Data and Information Set

The Health Plan Employer Data and Information Set (HEDIS) was created to provide employers with standardized information about health plan performance. The National Committee for Quality Assurance (NCQA), a private, not-for-profit organization created to assess the quality of managed care plans, developed HEDIS in collaboration with purchasers, health plans, and technical experts. NCQA is governed by a Board of Directors that includes employers, consumer and labor representatives, health plans, quality experts, regulators, and representatives from organized medicine. NCQA began accrediting managed care organizations (MCOs) in 1991. Although the accreditation program is voluntary, more than half of the HMOs in the nation are currently involved in the NCQA accreditation process.

NCQA released the first version of HEDIS 2.0 in November 1993, and it quickly became the most widely used performance measurement system among managed care plans, many of whom report HEDIS data to employer clients or use HEDIS data to inform their quality improvement efforts. Employers also adopted HEDIS to help guide their selection among health plans. Today, through employer initiatives, national magazines, and local newspapers many consumers receive HEDIS data in the form of health plan "report cards."

Consequently, NCQA released Medicaid HEDIS, a customized version of HEDIS that included measures relevant to the special populations served by the Medicaid program. In 1996, NCQA released HEDIS 3.0 to supplant both HEDIS 2.5 (a technical update to 2.0 released in 1995) and Medicaid HEDIS. HEDIS 3.0 enables both public and private purchasers to use the same performance measurement tool to evaluate plans, regardless of whether the plans serve commercial or public populations, an important step forward in the drive for accountability in health care.

Prior to version 3.0, HEDIS did not incorporate a standard tool for gathering information from plan enrollees about their satisfaction with health plan services. HEDIS 3.0 includes the new HEDIS 3.0 Member Satisfaction Survey, which provides comparable member satisfaction data from health plans across the country. The survey incorporates many questions from existing satisfaction surveys into a single instrument. For most of HEDIS, health plans report the data directly. However, NCQA requires that the new Member Satisfaction Survey be administered by a third-party organization. The survey is administered to plan enrollees via mail. It includes screening questions to confirm enrollee coverage and obtain sociodemographic data. It features questions to determine enrollees' satisfaction, as well as assess their health and functional status. In 1997, HCFA began to require Medicare managed care plans to report on performance measures from HEDIS 3.0 relevant to the Medicare managed care population, and participate in an independently administered Medicare beneficiary satisfaction survey, the Medicare version of CAHPS.

CONCLUSION

This chapter has reviewed some of the issues in the measurement and collection of patient satisfaction with or evaluation of care. Patient evaluation or satisfaction with physician or acute health care has been studied longer than any other service area. An increasing number of health programs are now involving patient assessments in their evaluation of health plans; others include patient evaluations of care in report cards or other tools to guide patient choice of health plan. Interest in the collection of consumer satisfaction and evaluation with health is peaking at this time for a number of reasons, including: (1) the recognition of subjective evaluations of care as an important indicator of care quality, (2) the growing interest in developing Total Quality Management (TQM) and quality improvement systems, and (3) increased competition among health care providers.

Chapter 8

Using Consumer Survey Results: Completing the Quality Cycle

We have spent an entire book thinking about how to hear the voices of consumers. From focus groups, to consumer logs, to large-scale surveys, we have emphasized the importance of creating mechanisms to hear what consumers have to say about their services. So now, after we have struggled with the seemingly endless stream of questions about the survey process, such as what instrument to use, how to select the sample, how to collect data, how and when to use proxies, and how and when to use consultants, we are faced with the $64,000 question: How do we use this stuff? After all, the reason for collecting consumer satisfaction information is to improve the quality of services. So how can these data be examined and then used to help an agency improve the quality of services. To this end, this chapter will present approaches to both analyzing and using data for quality improvement.

ANALYZING CONSUMER DATA

With the evolution of the personal computer, agencies, with a little help, can conduct a lot of the consumer satisfaction analysis. The initial analysis process would benefit from some outside consultation, but with good training we believe an agency can become almost independent on this task over time. It also may be the case that an agency would want to be part of a consortium of agencies in order to receive comparative data. Both approaches will be discussed in this section.

Internal Analysis

There are two ways for individual agencies to use consumer satisfaction results. First, agencies can establish a "gold standard", in which they have a specified goal for agency satisfaction results. For example, the agency objective might be to have 90% of recipients very satisfied with select services, or an average score of 4.5 out of 5 on a service satisfaction scale. Such service scores can also be examined over time. Collection of satisfaction data at 6- or 12-month intervals, for instance, could allow an agency to plot mean scores over time. Such an approach will allow agencies to develop benchmarks for continuous improvement.

The individual agency level strategy might also include a subgroup analysis, where satisfaction effects are examined for specific subcategories of consumers. For example, are consumers that experience higher levels of disability more satisfied with services? Do differences exist based on demographic characteristics, such as age, race, income status, or living arrangement? Could the agency be discriminating in any fashion, such that these differences might occur, or are there reasons for such differences to exist? These data will not answer this question definitely, but it will provide evidence about whether differences exist, in order for the agency to explore the quality question.

Case study or qualitative data can also be used to enhance the analysis. Case study information can be used to complement survey data, in an effort to help understand trends in satisfaction responses. In-person interviews provide agencies with the background material to understand why increases or declines in consumer satisfaction occur. For example, in a recent study of home care quality, a decrease in consumer satisfaction appeared to be linked to the agency financial constraints that caused them to cut back on the number of hours of service provided. Consumers felt that home care workers were pressed for time and this resulted in not only a decrease in frequency of hours spent helping, which had been anticipated, but a decrease in the perceived quality of the services provided. In-depth interviews, case studies, or focus groups are approaches described throughout the book that can be used to supplement process and outcomes data.

Comparative Analysis

A second major approach to analysis is for individual agencies to become part of a consortium of like agencies. Case management agencies, home care agencies, or other types of organizations delivering similar types of services to similar types of consumers can provide comparative data bases for each other. For example, how do the consumer satisfaction scores of your agency compare with the mean scores for similar agencies? In such a comparison we would typically compare the mean score for the individual agency to the overall mean of the comparison agencies. We would also give this mean score a percentile rank and provide the 25th and 75th percentile score rankings as a reference point for comparative purposes. Agencies can then compare their outcomes to others to gauge performance. Again, such data provide indicators of performance but should not interpreted as final outcomes. Additional factors, such as characteristics of clients, environment, resources available, culture, geographic region, and funding levels could effect consumer satisfaction outcomes. Statistical adjustments can be made in a comparative analysis to address some of these differences. For example, organizations that serve a more impaired population might report lower satisfaction scores, since we do know that respondents with higher levels of disability on average report lower consumer satisfaction scores. Typically, agencies will be part of a consortium for this type of analysis, so such adjustments will be made by the entity completing the overall analysis.

USING SATISFACTION DATA

Once agencies collect consumer satisfaction data, they are then in the position to combine such information with other data on program performance. Additional data elements could include the elapsed time from the initial call into the agency to the receipt of services, whether the clients met the enrollment characteristics for admission, or additional outcomes data such as mortality rates, program termination rates, hospital length of stay, or nursing home admission and discharge rates. These measures, along with satisfaction findings, combine to provide indicators of program quality.

Incorporating this type of information into agency operations represents the quality improvement process. Unfortunately most agencies spend the bulk of their time addressing the day to day problems, and precious little time examining performance data in the context of agency operations. These data can be useful in the improvement process in two major ways. First, to support ongoing improvement questions being examined by the agency. For example, an agency, unsure of whether their intake and assessment process was too burdensome for clients, was able to look at both the elapsed time data and consumer satisfaction information to make an assessment on program performance. Often, agencies will identify an area for improvement because of anecdotal information, without the benefit of systematic data about the size or nature of the problem. Having data available to inform the group addressing these types of questions, strengthens the agency's ability to come up with a productive solution. In some cases available data will be sufficient to address the question being studied, in others new data will be necessary.

As discussed in chapter 1, the quality improvement process relies on having information so that organizations can make good decisions about how to deliver care. In this example, without knowing how consumers feel about the services received and how long services take to be delivered it is very difficult to know if the process needs to be modified.

The second approach to using benchmark or comparative data is to use the information collected as a starting point for a review of program operations. For example, in examining comparative satisfaction data ,an agency finds that it has one of the lowest satisfaction scores of any of the comparative agencies in its group. These data can then spark a study of client and agency processes. Does the agency deliver services differently than the comparative agencies? Does it provide different amounts of services? Does the agency serve different types of clients? Does it serve a wider geographic area? Does the service planning or arrangement process differ from other agencies? Does the agency select providers in a different way? Does it reimburse providers in a different manner? What other differences exist that would explain these and other outcome differences? By addressing these types of questions the agency can then try to understand how operational differences effect client outcomes. Certain factors may be under the control of the agency, while others, such as the type of clients served clearly are not.

Understanding which factors influence satisfaction is critical in an agency's efforts to enhance its quality. In some comparative studies organizations can compare procedures and management operations across programs. For example, in a comparative analysis the agencies that score in the top 10% on consumer satisfaction could be examined in detail to see how their organizational structure or management-design or -techniques differ from those in the bottom quartile. Such a comparison can provide agencies with information on how to improve service delivery and represents a key element of the quality improvement process.

KEY STEPS FOR IMPLEMENTING A SUCCESSFUL CONSUMER SATISFACTION AND OUTCOMES STRATEGY

Now that we have laid out the key components to assessing consumer satisfaction, we are left with the final task of implementation. How can agencies or a group of agencies make this happen? In this final section, and in the best tradition of Letterman, we identify the top 10 key steps to implementing a successful strategy.

1. *Agreeing on agency commitment to hearing the voices of consumers.* We began this book by stating that the biggest challenge for any service agency is its ability to have a shared staff-commitment to hearing from consumers. Most organizations and individuals have mixed feelings about feedback. On one hand, we want to know what people think about how we perform. On the other hand,

we really only like to hear good things. The commitment to hearing what consumers have to say involves accepting the fact that in some cases consumers will not like how we deliver a service.

Most organizations make at least some attempt to assess consumer satisfaction. However, the vast majority are unsuccessful at this effort. The major reason is the lack of commitment or belief in the importance of consumer feedback. The importance of hearing from consumers must come from the top administrative staff of the agency if it has any chance of success. It also must permeate the entire organization. The health and long-term care fields contain many barriers to assessing consumer satisfaction. From the physical and mental frailty of many of the consumers, to the complexity of care and the lack of information about the delivery of services , there are numerous reasons why consumers voices are difficult to hear. Our experience in working with lots of agencies is that, unless there is a strong and unwavering commitment to involving consumers, there will always be many good reasons why consumes are unable to be involved.

2. *Agreement to change and improve the services based on consumer feedback and other process and outcome data.* The training of practitioners has long included an inherent conflict. That is, we want practitioners to be confident, in fact unwavering, about the services or treatment provided, even in instances where the treatment plan is less than clear. The outcome of that phenomena is that once we train and establish practice pattens for care, it is very difficult to change practice. Agency staff can be quick to dismiss consumer comments. In some instances consumer comments may be inaccurate or not helpful. But it is also the case that the consumers receiving services are in a very good position to communicate how a provider is doing. If agencies are going to ask consumers what they think about service delivery, it is essential that some recognition and some level of response be allowed. Asking consumers what they think and then ignoring their responses is worse then not asking at all.

Getting practitioners to agree on an improvement process that argues that you have to be willing to change the way services are provided based on data collected from and about consumers is a monumental challenge. Modifying long-established practice patterns, whether it be at the university where we developed our teaching techniques some time during the middle ages, or physician practice which took a long time to give up on blood-letting as an important intervention, requires practitioners to be willing to step back and reassess the delivery of services. In most agencies, the professional orientation that minimizes the importance of consumer feedback, dominates the organizational culture.

3. *Development of an overall strategy for type and frequency of information to be collected, including consumer satisfaction and other outcomes data.* Once agencies have made the commitment to collecting consumer satisfaction and outcomes information, it is essential to develop a strategy for data collection. Which data are to be collected routinely? Which outcomes are important to benchmark? How often does an agency want to collect data directly from consumers? When and how often are focus groups needed? What should the mix of data collection strategies look like? Because data collection and processing are expensive, agencies have to balance the need for information with cost. Thus, agencies consistently have to assess information needs for improvement in the context of service expenditures.

When we work with agencies, one of our first recommendations is to develop a data and quality strategy. This involves examining quality improvement goals in the context of agency characteristics including the budget, the number and type of clients served, computer capability and internal expertise, regulatory requirements, and experience in satisfaction and outcomes efforts. The plan or strategy requires the agency to think through both its resources and commitment to this effort. It also emphasizes the evolutionary nature of the process, highlighting the fact that all steps can not be completed immediately. We have not seen any agencies that were able to make significant progress without taking this strategic step.

4. *Development of a good system for processing client-level information.* As we visit agencies, the most common complaint we hear involves the workings of the management information system. Most organizations have developed at least adequate information processing systems in order to pay the bills, but very few have sys-

tems that meet other information needs. In most agencies, descriptive data on clients and how they have changed over time, detailed utilization and cost data, and information on expected outcomes of services are a rare entity.

Changes in both the computer industry overall and in software development for health and long-term care agencies has been astounding. The current generation of computers has enough processing power and memory to operate a typical agency system. As complicated as some of the hardware configurations can be, it is the software side that involves the most important decisions for agencies.

The software options for agencies are clearly a double-edged sword. On one hand, agencies now have more options available than ever before to choose from regarding how to configure and manage information. On the other hand, many agencies have purchased or had software custom-designed, that did not provide what was needed. There are a number of important questions that an organization needs to address in developing an information system that works. For example, will computers be used as part of service delivery, such as what is done by case management projects that now complete their initial assessments on laptops in the home of prospective clients. What type and frequency of analysis will be completed? What is the volume and type of data needed for quality improvement activities? Although developing a good management information system will most likely require external consultation, we feel very strongly that having staff ownership and direction is essential to ensuring a positive outcome of such an effort.

5. *Development of specific data collection tools and approaches.* One of the most common questions we're asked is how to select a specific instrument to assess consumer satisfaction. The major debate is between developing a new instrument that is tailored to your unique agency versus using an existing survey. A new instrument has the major advantage of being able to capture the nuances of a particular agency or program. The questions have the potential to demonstrate a better understanding of the program and could result in better data for quality improvement.

The use of an existing survey allows the agency to build on the work of others, using an instrument that has an established track record of success. Agencies are neither reinventing the wheel under this approach, nor are they risking the chance that the data does not meet acceptable standards of reliability.

Although each agency is unique, we typically recommend a hybrid approach to this problem. Under this strategy we primarily use existing instruments for surveying consumer satisfaction. However, we almost always develop new questions designed to capture the unique aspects of the program. The number of new questions might entail about 15% of the survey, while the remainder would come from established sources. We feel that such a strategy allows the agency to use acceptable instrumentation, while recognizing the unique aspects of the program or agency.

As we have discussed in earlier chapters, in each of the study areas there are a range of satisfaction surveys. Although we believe that some are better than others and have tried to point out that what is most important for agencies to recognize is that this is an evolutionary process and that the "perfect" instrument does not now exist. Agencies should in each of the service areas make an informed choice about what to use. However, it is critical to recognize that over time the measures and even which areas are most important may change. We have visited a number of agencies where the search for the perfect instrument has paralyzed the process. Thus, despite our commitment to quality management and the planning process associated with this technique, we feel that it is more important to get started, even if modification is necessary, than it is to agonize for years over the perfect tool—or, in the words of one of our colleagues, "Do something even if it's wrong!"

6. *Creating a mechanism for analyzing survey results and other information collected.* Once an agency has collected the necessary data and created a mechanism for storing and processing the information it needs an analysis plan. As noted earlier in this chapter, we believe that, over time, agencies can develop the capability to do most statistical analysis on its own. We do recommend the use of outside consultants in the initial stages and also encourage the use

of collaborative efforts. For instance, in many communities partnerships with universities provide a great opportunity for agencies to tap into research expertise and for the academic community to become more aware of practice issues and challenges.

Related to the earlier discussion about management information systems, one of the key challenges facing agencies is the inclusion of analytic capabilities in the information system software. When the typical agency has an information system designed and installed it does not specify analytic needs, and thus these requirements are almost always excluded from the system design. Agencies must have the ability to analyze data on a day-to-day basis if they are going to incorporate data use into the organizational culture.

7. *Linking information back to a quality improvement process.* Throughout the book we have emphasized how critical it is for agencies to identify a process through which they can link program data back to the delivery of services. Collecting consumer satisfaction and other outcomes data is somewhat atypical, and agencies that link this information back to service improvement is truly rare. Because agencies experience many competing demands on staff time and resources, developing a process that routinely links data to program management is critical if such data are going to improve services. We have identified several approaches that agencies use to link information to service improvement.

What is far more important, however, is that agencies build the expectation in to the organizational culture that quality improvement efforts will be linked to information.

8. *Modify type, amount, and mode of data collection to better meet service needs.* Figuring what data to collect is a difficult task for agencies. Once in place, the last thing any agency wants to think about is changing survey instruments or data collection forms. Although it is the case that such changes should not be made lightly, it is important that agencies recognize the need to modify data collection efforts over time. Using information as a means of improvement needs to be viewed as an evolutionary process. Areas of interest and importance will change over time. Just as it will be necessary to modify services based on experience, it will

also be necessary to modify the type, amount, and mode of data collection over time.

There are many lessons yet to be learned about the best way to collect information from consumers. In particular, we know very little about how such areas as ethnicity, race, gender, and geographic location will influence how consumers report about satisfaction. Even when we know that certain factors, such as education and income effect both consumer satisfaction and the responses older people provide, we know little about how to compensate for these challenges. We also have many lessons to learn about the optimum mode of data collection. We have presented the pros and cons of data collection options, but we still don't know what is the best approach to collect certain types of data for the diverse older population receiving services. There is much more to be learned about what to hear and how to hear the voices of consumers.

9. *Recognize that this process is a continuous one.* As we have emphasized continuously, the improvement process is constant. Whether we are delivering acute or long-term care services in a hospital, a nursing home, assisted living, or at home, improving care will never cease to be an issue. Technology and clinical skills continually change, as do consumers. Agencies, often especially very successful ones, have a tendency to believe that approaches that have worked in the past will clearly work in the future. Although many successful agencies will continue to enjoy success, it is not likely that they can continue to proper without changing and improving. There are countless examples of organizations that held on to their approach, long past the point of productivity or success from the view point of the consumer. Thus, what needs to be the hallmark of the agency is not what they do or make, but that they can continually make sure that what there doing is of high quality and meets the needs of its consumers.

10. *Give this book to a coworker.* We began this book by discussing the need for a shared commitment within the organization. In most agencies this will not happen quickly. There are typically three personality types with an organization. Group 1 will be on board, ready to make this happen. Group 2 is educable, but clearly needs training and support, and needs to recognize that senior manage-

ment thinks this is a good idea. Group 3 sees this as yet another hair-brain scheme that someone without enough to do has thought up for the agency. They are skeptical that this can work and wonder why we should be taking any time away from the delivery of services. Most of the people in this group will not be swayed until the agency can demonstrate some results. A few will never change their opinion about the importance of consumers or of the need to link data and improvement.

We recommend that you buy books for each group. We recognize that not all readers or employees will share the same zest that you do, but at least they will have the book.

Appendix

Selected Internet Resources for Consumer Satisfaction Efforts

Selected Internet Resources for Consumer Satisfaction Efforts

---

The Web sites listed below are intended to provide additional information, examples, and organizational support for consumer satisfaction efforts in health and long-term care. This is not an exhaustive list and as web sites change some of these resources may be incorrect or invalid.

QUALITY

http://www.jcaho.org.
Joint Commission on Accreditation of Healthcare Organizations. Academy of Healthcare Quality, general quality, and accreditation information. The National Library of Healthcare Indicators is a growing library of performance measurement systems and types of measures.

http://www.nahq.org.
National Association for Healthcare Quality. Publishers of the Journal of Healthcare Quality with some articles online at this Site. Also a resource list and links to other health care quality sites.

http://www.qmas.org/
Quality Measurement Advisory Service. Service to assist in measurement of health care quality. Links to tools, workshops, and other resources.

http://www.qualityhealth.org/
Foundation for Healthcare Quality. Sponsors programs on electronic commerce, quality measurement, and consumer affairs.

http://www.ahcpr.gov/qual/
Agency for Health Care Policy Research Quality Assessment. Links to outcome and performance measures such as Consumer Assessment of Health Plans Study (CAHPS) and Computerized Needs-Oriented Quality Measurement Evaluation System (CONQUEST). Also links to their research and publications.

EXAMPLES OF CONSUMER SATISFACTION APPROACHES

http://www.mhdi.org/
Minnesota Health Data Institute. Web site for performance outcome measurement in Minnesota for inpatient and outpatient health care. Includes patient survey information and reports. Good examples of consortium building to provide consumer satisfaction information and using focus group results to structure consumer satisfaction protocols.

http://www.nami.org/update/consumerstaff.html
National Alliance for the Mentally Ill. Description of a consumer satisfaction initiative to measure family and consumer satisfaction with behavioral health services.

http://www.pc.gov.au/research/commres/disabsvc/report.pdf
Review of Approaches to Satisfaction Surveys of Clients of Disability Services. Downloadable report provides good examples of several options for the Australian Government to implement a consumer satisfaction process for disability clients. Annotated bibliography of general and disability specific consumer satisfaction literature.

http://www.spry.org/
A Report on Customer Satisfaction Surveys in Nursing Homes from the Settling Priorities for Retirement Years (SPRY) Institute. Brief summary of a small-scale study of nursing home consumer satisfaction practices.

http://www.leadershipfactor.com
The Customer Satisfaction Network. Provides a forum for information exchange among persons interested in measuring customer satisfaction. Good brief overview of the measurement process and utilizing results.

http://customersat.com/
Internet survey experts. General overview of the satisfaction survey process along with sample questions.

http://atplus.com
Assessment Technologies Plus. Specialists in organizational assessments that create "strategic focus". Three tools measure quality within your organization, customer satisfaction, and employee satisfaction. Sample reports on the Web site provide good examples of satisfaction results analyses.

http://www.metrixmatrix.com/SScalc.asp
Online sample size calculator. Plug in an acceptable significance level and population size and it will calculate the number of people needed in a sample.

INSTRUMENTS

http://www.hcfa.gov/medicare/hsqb/oasis/oasishmp.htm
The purpose of this Site is to store and disseminate policy and technical information related to the Outcome and Assessment Information Set (OASIS) data set for use in HHAs (home health agencies). The information posted here is intended to assist HHAs, State agencies, software vendors, professional associations and other Federal agencies in implementing and maintaining OASIS.

http://www.ncqa.org/
National Committee on Quality Assurance, the accrediting entity for managed care plans. Information on managed care plans is provided to con-

sumers through this website. Questions from the Consumer Assessment of Health Plans (CAHPS) and Health Plan Employer Data and Information Set (HEDIS) are also available here.

CONSUMER INFORMATION AND ORGANIZATIONS

http://www.ncoa.org/consumerdirect/consumer_direct.htm
National Center for Consumer-Directed Services. A unit of the National Council on Aging dedicated to assistance and information with consumer-directed long-term care.

http://www.cinetserv.com/CMS/cmswebpage.pdf
Introductory brochure for the Consumer Medical Society, a membership organization for healthcare consumers.

http://www.cinetserv.com/CMS/cmswebpage.pdf
Consumer Health Information, Inc. Provides literature searches, consultation, and other healthcare information to consumers.

http://nccnhr.org/
National Citizens' Coalition for Nursing Home Reform, a consumer and advocacy group for people with long-term care needs.

http://www.ccal.org/
The Consumer Consortium on Assisted Living (CCAL) is a national consumer-focused organization that works collaboratively with a broad spectrum of people and organizations supporting quality assisted living as an essential option in long-term care.

ORGANIZATIONS IN AGING-, HEALTH-, AND LONG-TERM CARE

http://www.ahca.org/
American Health Care Association. Downloadable demonstration of their Facilitator Software which can be used as part of a quality improvement

system. Also a source of satisfaction surveys for nursing homes, assisted living facilities, and subacute facilities.

http://www.ache.org/
American College of Healthcare Executives. Publications and organization information.

http://www.aahsa.org/
American Association of Homes and Services for the Aging. National membership organization for not-for-profit providers of long-term care services. Provides accreditation to continuing care retirement communities.

http://www.nahc.org/
National Association of Home Care. Membership organization for home care and hospice providers.

http://www.acrweb.org/
Association for Consumer Research. Membership organization for professionals interested in psychological aspects of consumer behavior. Online, *Journal of Consumer Research.*

http://www.alfa.org/
Assisted Living Federation of America. Trade association serving the assisted living industry and their clientele. Information for consumers, researchers, providers, and others.

GENERAL INFORMATION ON AGING, HEALTH, AND LONG-TERM CARE

http://www.ahcpr.gov/
Agency for Health Care Policy Research. Information and publications on outcome measures and quality performance measures. Many publications are free and downloadable.

http://list.nih.gov/
National Institutes of Health Listserv. Center for professionals and researchers interested in long-term care and disability to communicate by subscribing to a variety of lists.

http://www.elderweb.com/index.html
Elderweb. 4,000 links to Internet sites on long-term care for caregivers, elders, professionals, and researchers.

http://www.nhirc.org/
National Health Information Resource Center. Clearinghouse for health and health care information. Discussion groups, research abstracts, consultants, and other information.

http://www.adldigest.com/
Aging-, Disability- and Long-Term Care. "The largest source of long-term care and disability information on the web". Subscription to an e-mail newsletter provides frequent updates on what's happening in the news, as well as resource lists to other Web sites on related topics, such as caregiving or housing.

http://pr.aoa.dhhs.gov/naic/
The National Aging Information Center (NAIC), operated by the U.S. Administration on Aging (AOA), is a central source for a wide variety of program- and policy-related materials and demographic and other statistical data on the health, economic, and social status of older Americans. Searchable databases, library resources, reports from AOA-funded projects, and links to other Web sites.

http://managedcare.hhs.gov/
This Site provides information relevant to researchers, policymakers, consumers, and advocates on a wide range of issues associated with managed care and disabilities. It is sponsored by the Office of the Assistant Secretary for Planning and Evaluation within the Department of Health and Human Services.

References

Abdellah, F., & Levine, E. (1957). Developing a measure of patient and personnel satisfaction with nursing care. *Nursing Research, 5*, 100–108.

Aharony, L. & Strasser, S. (1993, Spring). Patient satisfaction: What we know about and what we still need to explore. *Medical Care Review, 50*(1), 49–79.

American Association of Retired Persons. (1996). *Checkpoints for managed care: How to choose a health care plan*. Washington, DC: Author.

American Health Care Association. (1996). *Satisfaction Assessment Questionnaire*. Washington, D.C.: Author.

Anderson, E. W., & Fornell, C. (1994). A customer satisfaction research prospectus. In R. T. Rust & R. L. Oliver (Eds.), *Service quality: New direction in theory and practice*. Thousand Oaks, CA: Sage Publications.

Anderson, J. P., Kaplan, R. M., & DeBon, M. (1989). Comparison of responses to similar questions in health surveys. In R. Fowler, J. Floyd, Jr. (Eds.), *Health survey research methods: Conference proceedings*. Washington, DC: National Center for Health Services Research.

Andrews, F., & Withey, S. (1976). *Social indicators of well-being*. New York: Plenum Press.

Assisted Living Federation of America. (1998). *What Is Assisted Living?* [http:\\www.alfa.org].

Assisted Living Quality Coalition. (1998). *Assisted living quality initiative: Building a structure that promotes quality*. [http:\\www.alqual.org/news/assisted/toc.htm].

Attkisson, C. C., & Zwick, R. (1982). The client satisfaction questionnaire: Psychometric properties and correlation with service utilization and psychotherapy outcome. *Evaluation and Program Planning, 5*, 233–237.

Blalock, H. M. (1979). *Social statistics*. New York: McGraw Hill.

Blumenthal, D. (1996). Quality of health care: What is it? *New England Journal of Medicine, 335*(12), 891–893.

Bodenheimer, T. S. & Grumbach, K. (1995). *Understanding health policy: A clinical approach*. Norwalk, CT: Appleton & Lange.

Brambilla, D. J. & McKinlay, S. M. (1987). A comparison of responses to mailed questionnaires and telephone interviews in a mixed mode health survey. *American Journal of Epidemiology, 126*(5), 962–968.

Burwell, B. (1998). *Medicaid long-term care expenditures.* Lexington, MA: Systemics.

Cleary, P. D., & McNeil, B. J. (1988, Spring). Patient satisfaction as an indicator of quality care. *Inquiry, 25,* 25–36.

Cowles, C. M. (1995). *Nursing home statistical yearbook 1995.* Tacoma, WA: Cowles Research Group, Inc.

Crosby, P. B. (1979). *Quality is free: The art of making quality certain.* New York, NY: McGraw-Hill.

Cryns, A. G., Nichols, R. C., Katz, L. A., & Calkins, E. (1989). The hierarchical structures of geriatric patient satisfaction: An older patient satisfaction scale designed for HMO's. *Medical Care, 27*(8), 802–816.

Davies, A. R., & Ware, J. J. E. (1988, Spring). Involving consumers in quality of care assessment. *Health Affairs,* 33–48.

Davis, M. A., Sebastian, J. G., Tschetter, J. (1997). Measuring quality of nursing home service: residents' perspective. *Psychological Reports, 81*(2), 531–542.

Davis, D. & Hobbs, G. (1989, June). Measuring outpatient satisfaction with rehabilitation services. *Quality Review Bulletin,* 192–197.

Donabedian, A. (1966). Evaluating the quality of medical care. *Milbank Memorial Fund Quarterly, 44*(3), 166–206.

Donabedian, A. (1980). *Explorations in quality assessment and monitoring: Volume 1.* Ann Arbor, MI: Health Administration Press.

Edgman-Levitan, S. & Cleary, P. D. (1996). What information do consumers want and need? *Health Affairs, 15*(4), 42–56.

Eriksen, L. (1987, July). Patient satisfaction: An indicator of nursing care quality. *Nursing Management, 18*(7), 31–35.

Feasley, J. (1999). *Health outcomes for older people: Questions for the coming decade, Executive Summary.* Washington, D.C.: Institute of Medicine.

Folkes, V. S. (1994). How consumers predict service quality: What do they expect? In R. T. Rust & R. L. Oliver (eds.), *Service quality: New direction in theory and practice.* Thousand Oaks, CA: Sage Publications.

Gauthier, B. (1987). Client satisfaction in program evaluation. *Social Indicators Research, 19,* 229–254.

Geigle, R. & Jones, S. B. (1990). Outcomes measurement: A report from the front. *Inquiry, 27,* 7.

Geron, S. M. (1991). Regulating the behavior of nursing homes through positive incentives: An analysis of Illinois' Quality Incentive Program (QUIP). *The Gerontologist, 31,* 292–301.

Geron, S. M. (1995, March). *Utilizing elder focus groups to develop client satisfaction measure for home-based services.* Unpublished poster session at the

41st Annual Meeting of the American Society on Aging in Atlanta, Georgia, in March, 1995.

Geron, S. M. (1998). *The Home Care Satisfaction Measures (HCSM): Conceptual design and results of psychometric analyses* [Monograph]. Boston, MA: Boston University, School of Social Work.

Geron, S. M. (1998a). Assessing the satisfaction of older adults with long-term care services: Measurement and design challenges for social work. *Research on Social Work Practice, 8*(1), 103–119.

Gold, M. & Wooldridge, J. (1995). Plan-based surveys of satisfaction with access and quality of care: Review and critique. In *Conference Summary: Consumer survey information in a reforming health care system*. Rockville, MD: Agency for Health Care Policy and Research.

Gustafson, D., Gustafson, R., & Wackebarth, S. (1997). CHESS: Health information and decision support for patients and families. *Generations, XXI*(3), 56–58.

Gutek, B. A. (1978). Strategies for studying client satisfaction. *Journal of Social Issues, 34*(4), 44–56.

Guzman, P. M., Sliepcevich, E. M., Lacey, E. P., Vitello, E. M., Matten, M. R., Woehlke, P. L., & Wright, W. R. (1988). Tapping patient satisfaction: A strategy for quality assessment. *Patient Education and Counseling, 12*, 225–223.

Heath, J. B. H, Hultberg, R. A., Ramey, J. M., & Ries, C. S. (1984, Summer). Consumer satisfaction: Some new twists to a not so old evaluation. *Community Mental Health Journal, 20*(2), 123–134.

Herzog, A. R. & Rodgers, W. L. (1992). The use of Survey Methods in Research on Older Americans. In R. B. Wallace and R. F. Woolson (Eds.) (60–90), *The Epidemiologic Study of the Elderly*. New York: Oxford University Press.

Herzog. A. R. & Kulka, R. A. (1989). Telephone and mail surveys with older populations: a methodological overview. In Lawton, P. & Herzog, A. R. (eds.) 63–92. *Special Research Methods for Gerontology*. Amityville, NY: Baywood.

Hinshaw, A. S., & Atwood, J. R. (1982). A patient satisfaction instrument: Precision by replication. *Nursing Research, 31*, 170–191.

Holstein, M., & Cole, T. (1996). The evolution of long-term care in America. In R. Binstock, L. Cluff, & O. Meing, (Eds.), *The future of long-term care* (pp. 19–47). Baltimore, MD: John Hopkins University Press.

Hulka, B. S., Zyzanski, S. J., Cassel, J. C., & Thompson, S. J. (1970). Scale for the measurement of attitudes towards physicians and primary medical care. *Journal of Community Health, 1*, 256–275.

Hulka, B. S., Zyzanski, S. J., Cassel, J. C., & Thompson, S. J. (1971). Satisfaction with medical care in a low income population. *Journal of Chronic Diseases, 24*, 661–673.

Iglehart, J. K. (1992). The American health care system: Managed care. *New England Journal of Medicine, 327*(10), 742–747.

Iglehart, J. K. (1996). Role of the consumer. *Health Affairs, 15*(4), 7–8.

Jackson, J. S. (1989). Methodological issues in survey research on older adults. In Lawton, M. P. & Herzog, N. R. (Eds.). *Social Research Methods for Gerontology*. Amityville, NY: Baywood.

Kane, R. A., Kane, R. L., Illston, L. H., & Eustis, N. N. (1994, Fall). Perspectives on home care quality. *Health Care Financing Review, 16*(1), 69–89.

Kleinsorge, I. K. & Koenig, H. F. (1991). The silent customers: Measuring customer satisfaction in nursing homes. *Journal of Health Care Marketing, 11*(4), 2–13.

Komisar, H. L., Lambrew, J. M., & Feder, J. (1996). *Long-Term Care for the Elderly: A Chart Book*. Washington, D.C.: Institute for Health Care Research and Policy, Georgetown University.

Kraemer, H. C. & Thiemann, S. (1987). *How many subjects? Statistical power analysis in research*. Newbury Park, CA: Sage Publications.

Kramer, R. (1998). Industry snapshot. *Assisted Living Today, 6*(1), 38–47.

Kruzich, J., Clinton, J. F. & Kelber, S. T. (1992). Personal and environmental influences on nursing home satisfaction. *The Gerontologist, 32*(3), 342–350.

Larsen, D. L., Attkisson, C. C., Hargreaves, W. A., & Nguyen, T. D. (1979). Assessment of client/patient satisfaction: Development of a general scale. *Evaluation and Program Planning, 2*, 197–207.

Leape, L. L. (1994, December). Error in medicine. *Journal of the American Medical Association, 272*(23), 1851–1857.

Lebow, J. L. (1974, April). Consumer assessments of the quality of medical care. *Medical Care, 12*(4), 328–337.

Lebow, J. (1982). Consumer satisfaction with mental health treatment. *Psychological Bulletin, 91*(2), 244–259.

Lebow, J. L. (1983). Similarities and differences between mental health and health care evaluation studies assessing consumer satisfaction. *Evaluation and Program Planning, 6*, 237–243.

Linder-Pelz, S. (1982). Social psychological determinants of patient satisfaction: A test of five hypotheses. *Social Security Medicine, 16*, 583–589.

Linn, L. S. (1975). Factors associated with patient evaluation of health care. *Health and Society, Fall*, 531–548.

Lochman, J. E. (1983, Winter). Factors related to patients' satisfaction with their medical care. *Journal of Community Health, 9*(2), 91–109.

Locker, D., & Dunt, D. (1978). Theoretical and methodological issues in sociological studies of consumer satisfaction with medical care. *Social Science and Medicine, 12*, 283–292.

Lucas, M. D., Morris, C. M., & Alexander, J. W. (1988). Exercise of self-care agency and patient satisfaction with nursing care. *Nursing Administration Quarterly, 12*(3), 23–30.

MacKeigan, L., & Larson, L. N. (1989, May). Development and validation of an instrument to measure patient satisfaction with pharmacy services. *Medical Care, 27*(5), 522–536.

Magaziner, J. (1992). The use of proxy respondents in health surveys of the aged. (120–129) in Wallace, R. B. & Woolson, R. F. (eds.). *The Epidemiologic Study of the Elderly*. New York: Oxford University Press.

McArthur, J. H. & Moore, F. D. (1997, March). The two cultures and the health care revolution: Commerce and professionalism in medical care. *Journal of the American Medical Association, 277*(12), 985–989.

McGrew, K., & Quinn, C. (1997). Examining the effectiveness of telephone assessment and care planning for homecare services. *Generations, XXI*(1), 66–67.

McHorney, C. A., Kosinski, M., & Ware, J. E., Jr. (1994). Comparisons of the costs and quality of norms for the SF-36 health survey collected by mail versus telephone interview: results from a national survey. *Medical Care, 32*(6), 551–567.

Mehdizadeh, S., Applebaum, R., & Straker, J. (1996). Deja Vu All Over Again, Or is it?. *Nursing Home Use In The 1990's*. Scripps Gerontology Center. (Unpublished)

Meister, C., & Boyle, C. (1996). Perceptions of quality in long-term care: A satisfaction survey. *Journal of Nursing Care Quality, 10*(4), 40–47.

Merton, R. K. (1987). The focused interview and focus groups: continuities and discontinuities. *Public Opinion Quarterly, 51*, 550–566.

Miller, J. A. (1997). Studying satisfaction, modifying models, eliciting expectations, posing problems, and making meaningful measurements. In H. K. Hunt (ed.), *Conceptualization and Measurement of Consumer Satisfaction and Dissatisfaction*. Cambridge, MA: Marketing Science Institute.

Murer, M. J. (1997). Assisted living: The regulatory outlook. *Nursing Home Long Term Care Management, 46*(7), 24–27.

Norton, P. G., VanMaris, B., Soberman, L., & Murray, M. (1996). Satisfaction of residents and families in long-term care: 1. Construction and application of an instrument. *Quality Management in Health Care, 4*(3), 38–46.

O'Brien, K. (1993). Using focus groups to develop health surveys: an example from research on social relationships and AIDS-preventive behavior. *Health Education Quarterly, 20*(3), 361–372.

Oliver, R. L. (1977). A theoretical reinterpretation of expectation and disconfirmation effects on posterior product evaluation: experiences in the field. In Day, R. L. (ed.). *Consumer Satisfaction, Dissatisfaction and Complaining Behavior*. Bloomington, IN: Indiana University Press.

Packer, T., Race, K. E. H., & Hotch, D. F. (1994). Focus groups: a tool for consumer-based program evaluation in rehabilitation agency settings. *Journal of Rehabilitation, 60*(3), 30–33.

Parasuraman, A., Zeithaml, V. A., & Berry, L. L. (1985). A conceptual model of service quality and its implications for future research. *Journal of Marketing, 49*, 41–50.

Parasuraman, A., Zeithaml, V. A., & Berry, L. L. (1986). *SERVQUAL: A multi-ple-item scale for measuring customer perceptions of service quality.* Cambridge, MA: Marketing Science Institute.

Pascoe, G. C. (1983). Patient satisfaction in primary health care: A literature review and analysis. *Evaluation and Program Planning, 6,* 185–210.

Phillips, P. (1989). The search for quality. *Generations XIII*(1), 8–11.

Quine, S. & Cameron, I. (1995). The use of focus groups with the disabled elderly. *Qualitative Health Research, 5*(4), 454–462.

Reinharz, S. & Rowles, G. (1988). *Qualitative gerontology.* New York: Springer Publishing Co.

Riley, P. A., Fortinsky, R. H., & Coburn, A. F. (1992). Developing consumer-centered quality assurance strategies for home care: A case management model. *Journal of Case Management, 1*(2), 39–48.

Roberts, R. E., Pascoe, G. C., & Attkisson, C. C. (1983). Relationship of service satisfaction to life satisfaction and perceived well-being. *Evaluation and Program Planning, 6,* 373–383.

Ross, C. K., Steward, C. A., & Sinacore, J. M. (1995). A comparative study of seven measures of patient satisfaction. *Medical Care, 33*(4), 392–406.

Rust, R. T., & Oliver, R. L. (Eds.). (1994). *Service quality: New direction in theory and practice.* Thousand Oaks, CA: Sage Publications.

Scheer, J., & Luborsky, M. L. (1991). The cultural context of polio biographies. *Orthopedics, 14*(11), 1173–1181.

Simmons, S. F., Schnelle, J. F., Uman, G. C., Kulvicki, A. D., Kyong-OK, H. L., & Ouslander, J. G. (1997). Selecting nursing home residents for satisfaction surveys. *The Gerontologist, 37*(4), 543–550.

Spradley, J. P. (1980). *Participant observation.* Orlando, FL: Harcourt, Brace, Jovanovich.

Stamps, P. L., & Finkelstein, J. B. (1981, September). Statistical analysis of an attitude scale to measure patient satisfaction with medical care. *Medical Care, 19*(11), 1108–1135.

Strahan, G. (1997). Overview of nursing homes and their current residents: Data from the 1995 National Nursing Home Survey. *Advance Data, January 23. No. 280,* 1–10.

Straker, J. (1993). *Opportunities for resident control in long-term care institutions: A comparison across three types of facilities.* Unpublished dissertation, Northwestern University: Evanston, IL.

Uman, G. C. & Urman, H. N. (1997). Measuring consumer satisfaction in nursing home residents. *Nutrition, 13*(7–8), 705–707.

U.S. House of Representatives. (1997). *Medicare and health care chartbook.* Washington, D.C.: U.S. Government Printing Office.

United States General Accounting Office (GAO). (1996). *Skilled nursing facilities: Approval process for certain services may result in higher Medicare costs.* Washington, DC.: U.S. Government Printing Office.

Ware, J. E. & Snyder, M. K. (1975). Dimensions of patient attitudes regarding doctors and medical care services. *Medical Care, 13*(8), 669–682.

Ware, J. E. Jr. (1978). Effects of acquiescent response set on patient satisfaction ratings. *Medical Care, 16,* 327–336.

Ware, J. E. Jr., Davies-Avery, A., & Stewart, A. L. (1978). The measurement and meaning of patient satisfaction. *Health and Medical Care Services Review, 1*(1), 1–15.

Ware, J. E. Jr., Snyder, M. K., & Wright, W. R. (1976a). *Development and validation of scales to measure patient satisfaction with health care services. (Volume I of a final report) Part A: Review of literature, overview of methods and results from construction of scales. (NTIS No. PB288–329).* Springfield, MA: National Technical Information Service.

Ware, J. E., Snyder, M. K., & Wright, W. R. (1976). *Development and validation of scales to measure patient satisfaction with health care services. Volume I of a final report, part B: Results of scales constructed from the patient satisfaction questionnaire and other health care perceptions.* (NTIS No. PB288–330). Springfield, MA: National Technical Information Service.

Woerner, L., & Phillips, J. (1989). Client perspectives on quality care. *Caring, 8*(6), 47–51.

Woodruff, L. & Applebaum, R. (1996). Assuring the quality of in-home supportive services: A consumer perspective. *Journal of Aging Studies, 10*(2), 157–169.

Yi, Y. (1990). *A critical review of consumer satisfaction.* In V. A. Zeithaml (Ed.). *Review of marketing 1990.* Chicago, IL: American Marketing Association.

Zimmerman, D., Zimmerman, P., & Lund, C. (1996). The health care customer service revolution: The growing impact of managed care on patient satisfaction. Chicago, IL: Irwin Professional.

Zinn, J., Larizzo-Mourey, R. & Taylor, L. (1993). Measuring satisfaction with care in the nursing home setting: The nursing home resident satisfaction scale. *Journal of Applied Gerontology, 12*(4), 452–465.

Index